Tiny

TINY BUT MIGHTY
Life in the NICU & at home with
my Micro Premies

What I wish I had known
and how friends & family can help

JOANNA TACZANOWSKY

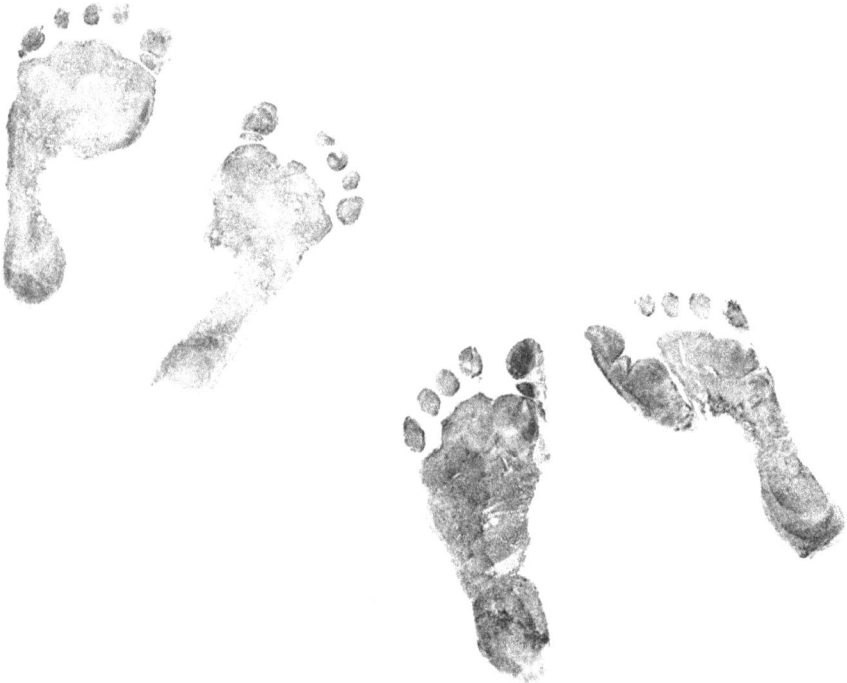

Tiny

Although the author and publisher have made every effort to ensure
that the information in this book was correct at press time, the author and publisher do not assume and hereby disclaim any liability
to any party for any loss, damage, or disruption caused by errors or
omissions, whether such errors or omissions result from negligence,
accident, or any other cause.

This book is not intended as a substitute for the medical advice of
physicians. The reader should regularly consult a physician in mat-
ters relating to his/her health and particularly with respect to any
symptoms that may require diagnosis or medical attention.

Cover design, book design and production by Jonathon Wolfer.
www.thelonewolfer.com

ISBN 978-0-9887989-4-6

For the amazing labor and delivery doctors, labor and delivery nurses, neonatologists, pediatric surgeons, neonatal nurse practitioners and neonatal intensive care nurses at Children's Memorial Hermann Hospital (Medical Center).

We would not be where we are today without you.
Dr. Charles Cox, Dr. Brian Jones, Dr. Cody Arnold,
Dr. See Wai Chang, Dr. Eric Eichenwald, Dr. Kathleen Kennedy,
Dr. Suzanne Lopez, Dr. Helen Mintz-Hittner, Tiffany Avery,
Lindsay Axford, Kim Cole, Priscilla Meyers,
Angie Morris, Beth Spencer, Vicki Simmering,
Kaitlin Perera & Dr. Amish Bhakta.

Tiny

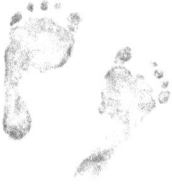

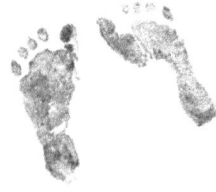

Forward

When my boys were born when I was only 24 weeks pregnant, I immediately purchased the few books I found on preemies and the Neonatal Intensive Care Unit (NICU) to try to prepare for the journey ahead. However, I found almost nothing that was helpful because none of the books went into detail about micro preemies (babies born before 26 weeks gestation), how different they are from premature babies (babies born before 36 weeks gestation), and what they might face during their stay in the NICU. Micro preemies can face very specific and very different obstacles compared to other premature babies. Most resources I found only offered a few sentences here and there about the hurdles specific to micro preemies. I was also immediately bombarded with questions from friends and family as to how they could help us. Looking back over the last year and a half I now have a new perspective on what we went through and how I could have better asked for help.

Having a baby in the NICU can be a terrifying roller coaster ride. Now on the other side, I thought sharing my story might be of benefit for someone just beginning their journey. If I had found a resource to provide my family, I think they could also have had an easier time supporting us through our time in the NICU and beyond.

Tiny

Tiny

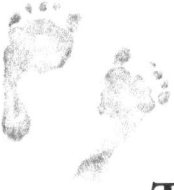

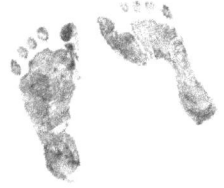

The Start of Our Journey

FINDING OUT I WAS PREGNANT WITH TWINS was one of the most exciting days of my life. My pregnancy began with In Vetro Fertilization (IVF) because conceiving without it was statistically not possible for my husband and me. We had been told there was a 30% chance that both embryos we transferred during our first round would implant, so it was not exactly a shock to find I was carrying twins, but it was thrilling. I had assumed that giving birth to two baby boys would be a day filled with excitement, joy and happiness (as well as pain and all the other not so jubilant things all your friends tell you giving birth will entail). I had been assured by my obstetrician/gynecologist (OB/GYN) that if both boys were head down I could try for a vaginal birth, but if one or both were breech (feet down) or sideways (transverse) I would have a Cesarean section (C-section). Statistically, most twins are born by C-section, so that is what we were preparing for, while hoping for a vaginal birth. I told my OB/GYN early on I wanted to exclusively breastfeed, and his response was "It's good to have goals." He certainly did not want to dissuade me, but he was familiar with the difficulties of breastfeeding one baby, let alone two, and did not want me to be crushed if that were unable to happen. Now I appreciate, and borrow, his response often. It is great to have goals, lofty goals even, but reality is often very different than what you imagine so it is also good to prepare to go with the flow.

Looking back now, the emotion that I associate most strongly with giving birth to my boys is terror. I do not like to think about it much, to be honest. My birth experience turned out to be nothing like I had imagined and nothing like I have ever seen on T.V. or heard about from friends or family. I had not anticipated any of what actually happened. Everything until week 23 of my pregnancy was completely normal. Besides my hips aching, beginning about week 12, which made sleeping for more than an hour at a time impossible, and some slight dehydration and false back labor, everything had gone completely according to plan. Even after the false back labor everything looked perfect and normal and no one anticipated seeing me in the hospital for many months to come. However, I woke at 4 am on Wednesday, April 24, 2013, to my water breaking. I was only 23 weeks and 6 days pregnant. It felt exactly how I would have imagined my water breaking would feel, but I tried to convince myself otherwise. I was absolutely terrified of what my water breaking would mean. After a few minutes my husband and I faced reality and got in the car headed for the emergency room.

My OB/GYN had told me during my first prenatal appointment that my local hospital, where he delivers, was prepared for babies born 26 weeks and later. Babies born before that would be medevacked downtown to the affiliated children's hospital with a NICU prepared to give care for more premature babies. Before my OB/GYN arrived at the emergency room, the E.R nurse summoned a NICU nurse who spoke with my husband and gave him a chart that detailed, for various gestational ages, the percentages of live births, major developmental and physical delays and minor developmental and physical delays. While realistic, the information was not delivered with the best bedside manner; she went into how their little organs, eyes, brains, etc. were not very developed at this stage and that we should expect everything that came along with that. I am glad I could not hear their conversation because my husband told me much later on that she had basically told him that probably neither baby would survive, but if they did, severe physical and developmental consequences would follow. I am very thankful for my ignorance, because for some reason it did not occur to me that either of the babies would not survive. Shortly after, my OB/GYN came in with the same degree of optimism and said that 24 weeks was almost the lowest limit of viability, but that if we were going to have a fighting chance the boys would need to be born downtown at the Children's Hospital. There was too much shock for me to think about what was happening in more than just the present moment. I am a pragmatic person to begin with and I kicked into high gear of "This is what has happened…let's deal with it" without thinking about what might be on the horizon.

After confirming that my water had indeed broken, giving me the first of two steroid shots to help with the babies' lung development, starting an IV in each hand for antibiotics and medication to try to stop labor, and inserting a catheter (never a good sign when the nurse tells you "We usually do this after an epidural, so brace yourself"), my OB/GYN deemed me stable enough to be transported downtown by ambulance to Children's Memorial Hermann Hospital. Later down the road my husband and I would realize how lucky we were that I was stable enough to be transported downtown before the babies were born and had not had to deliver at one hospital and have the babies flown to another. While I rode in the ambulance downtown to a hospital I had never been to, my husband drove home to get the dog settled for the day and then drove to meet us at the hospital.

Upon arriving, I was admitted and assessed by doctors, nurses, and medical students, all with the same plan of stopping labor and monitoring the babies. When we learned that I did not have to give birth immediately just because my water had broken, I told all of them that I planned on being there a long time without delivering. I was told there was a woman down the hall whose water had broken 6 weeks previously and she was nearing 35 weeks. That was very uplifting and I decided that is what I would do. When shift change came a few hours later and the incoming labor and delivery nurse introduced herself with "I'll be your delivery nurse today," the outgoing nurse corrected her "Nope, she's going to be here for a while." Everyone's primary concern was getting the babies to stay inside for as long as possible.

I was only contracting about 4 times every hour, showed no signs of infection, and was not in any real pain. Things looked positive. As the day wore on my parents became concerned I had not been returning phone calls or texts. My husband and I finally told our parents and a few close relatives what had happened and what our plan was. Of course everyone was very concerned and wanted to know how they could help. We assured everyone there was nothing to be done but wait. Our neighbor had agreed to let our dog in and out that day and my husband's company generously offered to put him up in a hotel down the street. We could not think about much of anything at the time, let alone how others could help us. Since we had both been up since 4 am, there was not much to do but hang out, try to nap, try to help the nurse reposition the monitor over each baby (because one or both babies would move and cause the heartbeat to become too faint to pick up), and try to keep track of the various antibiotics and medications that were switched in and out of my two IVs.

During day two in the hospital, I was given the second of the two steroid shots that help with lung development. Ideally the two shots are given 24 hours apart, but they can be given 12 hours apart. It was great we had made it 24 hours. Unfortunately we were also told that, although there is much research touting the steroid's ability to help lung development when babies are delivered before full term, not much research exists on how helpful the medication is when babies are born close to 24 weeks. The hope was that the steroids help the babies' lungs, but it has not been studied with micro preemies as it has with preemies. Things were going so well that it looked as though I would not give birth imminently and I was moved from the labor and delivery room to another room where I could be monitored. My catheter was removed for me to use the restroom on my own. I was allowed liquids for the first time since being admitted, which was great since I had not eaten anything since dinner the night before because doctors feared I would need a C-section.

* * * * *

Being admitted for preterm labor is very scary. A lot of information is being thrown at you and all you can think about is "Is my baby going to be okay?" Do not be afraid to ask a lot of questions about you and your baby. If labor and delivery nurses or doctors cannot answer all of your questions, they can call in NICU nurses and neonatologists who can. Having a significant other or a friend with you who can help keep track of your questions and the answers is very helpful.

Your job while in the hospital is to relax and keep the baby growing. Everything else can wait and can be taken care of by someone else.

* * * * *

Family and friends can ask about visiting policy and can bring other children to visit you, if possible. Sometimes a hospital's visitor policy changes during flu season. While in the hospital with preterm labor, there is a lot of monitoring and a lot of unending hours just lying in bed. Every hour the baby is able to grow and develop inside you saves many NICU days.

* * * * *

If you end up in the hospital for a prolonged period, friends and family can send books, a journal, DVDs or anything to keep you occupied (knitting, crocheting, Sudoku, crosswords, a laptop, e-reader, sketch book, and, believe it or not, even coloring books and crayons are all things other moms I know have done) to help pass the hours.

SINCE WE BEAT THE ODDS AGAINST DELIVERING within 24 hours, we were hopeful I would continue for weeks. Unfortunately things changed that afternoon when I got up to use the bathroom. The nurse asked if I was sure I did not feel anything unusual and I assured her I just needed to use the restroom. When I sat down, I felt as if I had to urinate but could not. I instinctively reached down to feel something I knew was not right. It was a baby's head. I called to the nurse and she and my husband helped me back into bed, as a doctor was immediately alerted and ran in. I guess it was a doctor; I honestly have no real memory of who did what next because it was then a blur of activity around me. I was quickly wheeled on the bed down the hall to a surgical suite that instantly filled with labor and delivery and neonatal doctors and nurses.

I did not realize my husband had left until he returned and was told to sit by my head. The anesthesiologist introduced himself, but since there was no time to offer any kind of pain medication, I assume now he was there just in case I needed to be put under general anesthesia for some reason. Both the babies had been head down, but if all of a sudden I had to deliver and one or both moved position I imagine I would have been given general anesthesia and a C-section. The most vivid part of being in the operating room was the pain from one nurse holding a monitor over Baby A (whose water had broken and whose head I had felt) and another nurse holding a monitor over Baby B. The monitors were plastic disks snugly belted against my belly, but because both babies were positioned head down on my bladder and I had not been able to use the restroom I was unbelievably uncomfortable with a full bladder that was now being even more compressed with babies and with monitors. That discomfort was infinitely worse than the contractions I was still feeling only a few times an hour. The doctor told me we were not waiting for a contraction to push (like you see on T.V.) but rather the nurse encouraged me into position to begin pushing the baby out immediately. I tried my best to do what they were telling me, regardless of how foreign and incorrect everything felt. Luckily it did not take more than 2 pushes and Baby A was born at 4:26 pm on April 25, 2013, only 36 hours after his water broke. After baby A was born, the neonatal transport team took him to be stabilized. Apparently my husband looked so shocked at the state of our child that the attending doctor had to ask him if he was alright. He was, but he felt crushed at the sight of our baby in that state.

The NICU transport team worked on the baby as my husband looked on. The attending doctor then instructed the resident how to tie off Baby A's umbilical cord and tuck it back in my uterus with the placenta as to have as little disruption as possible in order to try to hold off Baby B's delivery. At the time I had not known it was possible to deliver one baby and not the second. In fact, I had asked one of my nurses the day before if that was possible and she had said that it was not; if they had to deliver one baby, they would deliver the other. I was lucky in that they were both head down and I could deliver only the baby whose water had broken. If they were both feet down, I would have needed a C-section and both babies would have been born. It was a relief to be told in the operating room that there was a chance Baby B could stay inside longer to continue to develop. Once the doctor finished cleaning everything up, he graciously put in a catheter to relieve my bladder (my second unmedicated catheter). A moment later a transport nurse wheeled the baby in a transport isolette by me and said "Your husband tells me this is Charles." Without thinking I replied "No, I think it's Henry." My husband and I had recently agreed on names but had not reached the point of discussing which baby was which. At that moment I realized I had been thinking of the baby on my left as Henry and the baby on my right as Charles. My husband would have agreed to just about anything at that point so there was no argument from him. Henry James had officially entered the world weighing 1 pound, 5 ounces and measuring 12 inches long. The whole ordeal felt as though it took mere seconds. In reality, I do not think we were in the operating room more than a few minutes. Soon I was wheeled back to the labor and delivery room. The goal had changed. Now I told everyone I was going to keep this second baby in for as long as possible.

My husband was able to go to the NICU later on, after all the important things the NICU nurses needed to do to our baby had been completed, and he was able to bring back a photo on his cell phone. It was the second glimpse of my tiny baby and it was pretty frightening, to be honest. He was very red, he had a ventilator tube coming out of his mouth, his diaper appeared to swallow half his body, he had a mask over his eyes to protect them from the UV light over him (for jaundice), he had heart monitors taped to his torso, a monitor wrapped around his foot, and cords coming out from his umbilical cord. He looked unbelievably tiny. I did not think to count fingers. I forgot to count toes. All the things that T.V. shows demonstrate moms and dads doing to their perfect newborns did not even occur to me. Even if it had, we could not really have done any of it; we could not see all of him that well to make sure everything was there and perfect. I really just wanted to see him. I also wanted to keep Baby B in as long as possible. For the time being, it was back to lying in bed, waiting for time to pass, and telling everyone I was planning on being there a long time to give this baby still inside me the best chance I could.

We called the few family and friends who knew where we were and told them Henry had been born. They were very somber phone calls and lacked the typical joy and excitement you would think about when calling your parents to tell them their first grandchild had been born. Everyone was unbelievably scared that he had been born and of what that would now mean for his survival. We also told them about the plan that involved me staying in the hospital on bed rest in order to delay Baby B's birth as long as possible. We were just beginning to absorb our new situation.

Things had barely calmed down a few hours later when I was allowed to drink some broth and told to rest. After a few more hours passed and half the night had been wasted not sleeping through the mere 5 or so contractions I was having an hour, my husband suggested I ask a nurse if I could have a mild pain killer. This wonderful nurse took a hard look at me and said she wanted the doctor to come take a peak first. The resident came in and said she wanted to take a look at my cervix visually before giving me anything. She was not going to do a physical exam to feel how dilated I was because she did not want to introduce anything more that could cause infection. It was crushing to hear a few seconds later that she could see the baby's bag of water was bulging. It was so disappointing and unexpected. I had not felt anything different since returning from the surgical suite, and I had no idea things were changing so rapidly. I felt as though all my hopes were again taken away.

Since I had not felt anything different over the previous hours, we were completely caught off guard that this baby was coming now. The process of turning the room over from labor to delivery began. I was given an epidural, at the attending's request. He relayed to the resident that he was not sure how difficult or painful it would be to deliver Baby A's placenta after Baby B was born, and he certainly did not want to have to rush to the operating room again in order put me under general anesthesia to do that after the baby was born. After the room and team were ready and the resident broke my water, everything came to a stop. I was still only contracting every 15 minutes or so and was unsure what to do next since I had not received an instruction. I asked what I was supposed to do and the resident told me they were waiting for a contraction so that I could push, this being slightly less of an emergency delivery. It seemed to me as though that was a waste of time, and since I had already delivered a baby without contractions I asked if I should just try to push. Everyone seemed to think that was an okay idea so I did. Six pushes later Baby B was out. He actually shocked everyone and came out with a tiny cry. Charles 'Chuck' David was born at 3:33 am on April 26, 2013, weighing 1 pound, 8 ounces and measuring 12 inches long. He was born 11 hours after his brother.

The NICU transport team took over in the adjoining room and he was whisked upstairs to the NICU as soon as they were finished preparing him for transport. Both placentas were then seamlessly delivered by another resident (resident or student? I was not sure as it seemed like a lot of people in the room were being instructed what to do. That is how it can be in a teaching hospital). I felt like saying "Good job!" when she delivered the placentas. It was obvious it was her first time. Later I realized it was probably the first time for everyone in the room to be present for a delayed delivery like mine, since delivering one twin much before the second is not common at all. Between two states, medical centers reported 14 cases in 12 years. It was a very rare beginning to the boys' lives and, frankly, a very sad ending to my pregnancy. But with it, my pregnancy ended and our NICU journey began.

I was very lucky and had no complications after delivery. Other than a huge amount of swelling from the multiple large I.V. bags of antibiotics, medications to stop contractions, and medication to help my uterus retract after giving birth, I felt fine. Everything was normal for having given birth to two babies. I was finally able to eat solid food for the first time in a few days, which made me feel somewhat more normal.

Within two hours the recovery nurse conveyed to the lactation department that I was planning on pumping and ultimately breastfeeding; therefore, in the early hours of the morning someone brought me a breast pump and briefly instructed me how to use it. I had dreamed of being able to breastfeed, but for now this was all I could offer the boys. I began to pump immediately using the breast pump and the tiny plastic containers I was given. A few hours later I was given the okay to be wheeled in a wheelchair to the NICU for the first time and I had a tiny amount of colostrum to bring with me. My husband had been able to take one photo in the delivery room while the neonatal transport team was getting Chuck ready for his transport isolette. That was the only picture I had seen of him all morning since the NICU team had to work on him to get all the initial cords and wires in and on him. All I had seen of him was that he was very red and very swollen. He had a continuous positive airway pressure (CPAP) mask covering his whole face because, amazingly, for a few hours he had been breathing well enough not to require intubation. He had all the same monitors, all the same cords, and all the same paraphernalia as Henry had attached to his tiny body. I was anxious to see where Henry had been taken care of and who had been caring for my baby for the last almost half a day and also to see Chuck. As soon as we were allowed, my husband showed me the way to the NICU.

Going to the NICU for the first time is a very scary experience. Pretty much everything about it is awful. No matter how big your baby is when they are born, it is never a good thing when they have to go to the NICU. It is awful that your baby is sick or has a condition requiring them to be there. It is awful that babies are born so early that they have to be kept alive there. It is awful that you have to remember to wash your hands every time you touch your phone or camera or anything from home that has germs on it before touching your baby again. It is awful that you have to use pump after pump of hand sanitizer to the point that your hands get red and crack and bleed every time you visit. It is awful that the sounds of beeps and buzzers and machines are constantly going off indicating a baby is having a problem. It is awful that there are up to 6 babies in one large room sharing nurses and doctors and you never feel completely alone with your baby. It is awful that not every baby is going to get healthy and leave to go home. It is awful to see and hear mothers and fathers who at that very moment are saying goodbye to a baby. It is all just awful. Everything is awful. Everything is awful except the people. Those doctors and nurses and technicians who are there working tirelessly for all the babies, they are the saving grace of the NICU.

*****

I felt every emotion when the boys were born. I was excited to see them, I was utterly sad they were going to need to stay so long in the hospital, and I was so scared for them. Not having been able to touch them, let alone hold them and bond with them, I also felt pretty disconnected from them. I think there is no emotion that would not make sense to feel in that situation. It may help to talk with someone about your feelings, such as a close friend or a family member, but I felt that if I started talking I would fall apart. Most women I have talked to have a major breakdown or two (or lots) while their baby is in the NICU. I did not happen to have that experience or think it would helpful to me to let it all out, but everyone is different. I decided that I needed to move forward and take every day or every hour at a time. For me, it became more helpful to talk to the NICU nurses than to friends or family who could not fully grasp the situation in which I was. The nurses who deal with sick and fragile babies day in and day out, even though they may not have been in your shoes as a parent, can be very understanding when it comes to what you are going through. At any rate, know that anything you are feeling is valid.

* * * * *

Who should you tell that your baby has arrived so early or so sick? There is no right answer. Some parents wait until the baby is doing better before announcing. Some announce immediately. We decided to wait because we thought it would be too hard for us to explain what had happened and to relay all that the boys were going through when the boys' future was so uncertain. Frankly, we wanted to let some time pass until we were surer we would be announcing our babies' births and not also their deaths. It was very uncertain what our outcome would be and therefore we only told immediate family and a few friends when the boys were born.

* * * * *

About 50% of babies born at 24 weeks survive. Of those, 30-40% will develop normally and not suffer any major health concerns or disabilities, 20-35% will have a major disability (Cerebral Palsy, severe intellectual impairment, hearing or vision problems), and 25-40% will have minor disabilities (mild visual impairment, mild Cerebral Palsy, asthma, chronic lung disease). Both our boys were very sick and their situation very serious. This was part of the reason we wanted to wait until we had a better grasp on what their future might look like before we sent out their birth announcements.

* * * * *

It may be very difficult to know what to say to someone whose baby is born too early or when a baby's birth is both a happy and also very scary event. Someone at my husband's office, after he returned to work the Monday following the boys' births, said "Congratulations…and I'm so sorry" which I felt was totally appropriate. Simply acknowledging that you are sorry to hear that the baby was born so early and offering your support goes a long way.

* * * * *

It is not helpful to hear "Everything will be alright." Simply put, as many cases as there are where everything does turn out alright, there are as many cases where everything does not. Premature babies are vulnerable to so many things that it is not helpful to tell parents that you are sure everything will be okay, because it very well may not be. The few people who told us "I'm sure everything is going to be just fine" had the best intentions in the world, but I always felt like replying "No, you don't know that, no one can know that; everything might not be okay." It is very difficult for most people to understand how sick babies can be and how uncertain the future can be.

* * * * *

We were offered many stories of babies born to friends or to people that our family knew, or knew of, who were born early and are now doing great. We got a lot of these stories. People wanted to make us feel better by telling us every story they could about a baby who was born as early as ours and who was now a thriving toddler or adult. For us, that was not as comforting as it was intended to be. While it is wonderful that those stories had a happy ending, and we know they were shared with the most sincere intention to make us feel better, we were very unsure of whether or not our boys' story would end happily. Yes, we wanted to stay positive, but we also wanted to be realistic. Our babies had a 50/50 chance of living. That is very stark. Of course there are lots of brilliant stories about babies who defied the odds and surprised everyone and turned out wonderfully. However, given the statistics, there are just as many stories of babies who did not make it. People usually do not share those as readily and certainly would not be offering them up to parents of babies born prematurely. It is a fine line to walk; while everyone wants to be as supportive as they can be we also wanted to be realistic. The nurses and doctors were great at keeping us both positive and realistic. They made sure we were aware of everything that was going well and yet balanced that with reminding us how very sick our babies were.

* * * * *

It was very important to us that family and friends simply acknowledged our precious babies. That may be the most helpful thing you can do for parents of a baby in the NICU. While you may not want to send a "Congratulations on your baby's birth!" balloon centerpiece, it is appropriate to acknowledge the birth. A simple card letting us know that someone was thinking of us and our boys and hoping or praying that they were doing better every day meant a lot.

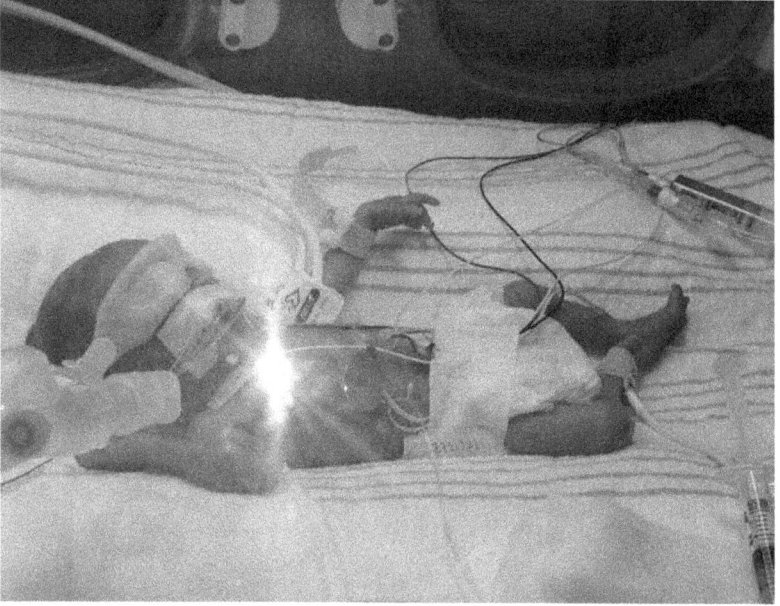

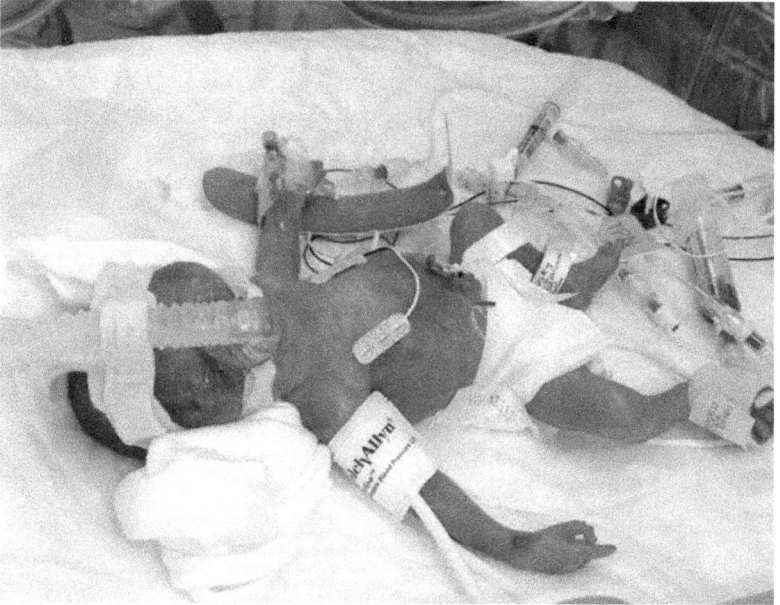

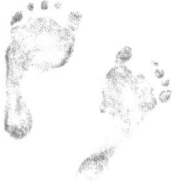

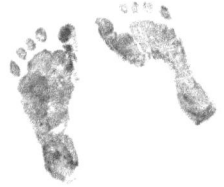

Not the Birth You Planned For

LOOKING BACK, WHILE I WAS IN THE HOSPITAL before the boys were born, I did not really have time to be fearful of their birth. I was so sure I could make it days, weeks, months before giving birth after my water broke that I did not spend any time worrying about all the things that could go wrong if they were born early. In hindsight I am not sure what good that would have even done. I am glad I can say I could not have done anything more to prevent their premature birth. I did everything I was told. I did not drink any caffeine when I was pregnant, I ate the healthiest I ever had, I did not over-do it (I was working from home on my couch or not working at all), I had followed the advice given in a highly respected book for multiples pregnancy and I had gained the 25 pounds by week twenty as is advised-even while being nauseous every day, I had gotten the okay from both my OB/GYN and my high risk OB/GYN to fly to attend my baby shower. No one had any concerns about me or the flight or the boys. Some premature labors can be explained by infection or trauma but mine was one of those completely unexplained premature labors. So I am glad I did not spend time worrying about what could have been or what should have been or what I should have done differently because that would not affect what happened once the babies arrived. I also do not like to think about the actual births for a long time. Frankly, I still do not like to think about them in detail. Being rushed to an operating room when you are 24 weeks and 1 day pregnant is not something I think I will ever want to think about for long. It is too emotional. It happened. I moved on.

* * * * *

The book I followed was "When You're Expecting Twins, Triplets, or Quads: Proven Guidelines for a Healthy Multiple Pregnancy, 3rd

Edition" by Barbara Luke. Among other helpful information, it recommends gaining 25 pounds by week 20 (of the typically recommended 40 pounds to be gained with twins) because after week 20 and towards the end of pregnancy it can be more difficult to gain weight. Our neonatologists and NICU nurses thought my early weight gain may have been responsible for the boys' borderline heavy birth weights, compared to other 24 week twins they had handled.

OF COURSE IT WAS EXTRAORDINARILY DISAPpointing to be discharged 4 days after I was initially admitted, 2 days after Chuck was born, since I had been hoping to last so much longer still pregnant in the hospital. To say it was very hard to leave the boys in the hospital and drive 45 minutes away from them is an understatement. But it was also comforting to be back in my own home and be away from IVs and nurses (as nice as they are) coming in to take my vitals every few hours, use my own shower, open my own fridge, and pet my own dog. Yet as soon as I took a moment at home to breathe, I immediately wanted to be back at the hospital with the boys. That feeling did not ever really go away. Every minute I was home I wondered how the boys were doing, wanted to be at the hospital and felt like, as their mother, I should be there and not at home while someone else took care of my babies. And every minute I was at the hospital I wanted to be home. It was a hard yo-yo. But people at the hospital were there to help with that.

Before I was discharged a labor and delivery doctor explained all the postpartum things that were normal. Since I had never given birth before, there was a lot I did not know. Pass a plum-sized blood clot? Normal. Bigger? Not. Who knew!? Both the discharge doctor and my discharge nurse were pleased I did not need any medical help with pain management since I was up and about showering and visiting the NICU as soon as I was given the okay. Luckily I was not really in pain. I think too much was going on and I needed to do other more important things than to sit down and think about how I felt. I would have almost felt guilty to take pain medication. My boys were struggling in the NICU and I needed medication to ease my pain? That would have been very difficult for me and I think it would be for a lot of moms. But it should not be. I needed to be healthy and strong for the months ahead, as do all parents of babies in the NICU. In case no one has ever told you, giving birth hurts. Unmediated emergency birth can be especially difficult; and unmedicated emergency birth plural even more so. Also C-sections (so I have been told and can imagine) are major surgery and can be extremely difficult to recover from. Nothing is wrong with realizing you are in pain and taking advantage of what is available to you for pain management. You cannot be there for your baby if you take on too much and push too hard and develop a complication after birth.

I also saw a social worker before I was discharged. I did not even know hospitals have social workers. She was unbelievably caring, knowledgeable, and helpful both at discharge and in the months to come. The packet of information she had for me contained everything from how to call Medicare (which the boys qualified for based on their low birth weights alone) to how to arrange for a parking contract in the parking garage across the street from the hospital (because otherwise we would have paid $9 a visit, twice a day, every day, which would have been $2,412 instead of the $750 we paid over the course of the boys' NICU stay) to what to watch for in terms of postpartum depression to phone numbers for helpful departments within the hospital. It was full of very helpful information. Of course I was not ready to absorb it all in the moment as I was being discharged, but I highlighted some information I thought I would need and wrote some notes and put the packet away to pick up later when I needed it. She also told me she had visited the NICU and thought the boys were doing as well as could be hoped. It was obvious how well suited for her job she was and how much she cared about both my babies and about me and how she was there to offer support and help in any way she could. She cared about moms, like me, who were all of a sudden thrown into a situation in which they had never been and wanted to help make it more manageable. I also got a visit from the hospital's March of Dimes® representative. She had some personal items such as shaving cream and a razor. She also had information about the March of Dimes® and how they support premature babies. She was helpful in the months to come by bridging the gap between my OB/GYN and the hospital, informing him of my discharge and also keeping him up to date a few times about the health of the boys.

* * * * *

It takes a moment to feel that this birth experience that you have planned for or thought about (or in some cases experienced before) is really over. Since statistically the majority of twins are born by C-section, I had assumed that was how I would give birth. I had not really thought much about a vaginal delivery and certainly not a natural one. Since we were fairly sure these would be our only children, it took a minute for it to sink in that my birth experience was over forever. I think it is normal that sadness accompanied that for me.

* * * * *

Information for anything from finding food at the hospital to parking to insurance to post-partum care can be found through your social worker, discharge nurse or NICU nurse. They themselves may not have the answer but can point you in the direction of the person who can help you.

* * * * *

Giving birth by C-section and then having to deal with a baby in the NICU is certainly a lot to handle both physically and emotionally. Since a C-section is major surgery, certain physical restrictions follow afterwards to ensure that your body can heal properly. Driving and walking long distances may be difficult, or prohibited for a period of time. If a friend or family member lives close enough and is available, an offer to drive to and from the hospital so mom can visit her baby might be very helpful. Also, the hospital can arrange a wheelchair for your use when visiting your baby. You have to remember all you are doing to heal as well, and surprising accommodations can be made if you simply ask.

* * * * *

Bring home everything the hospital offers you - you never know what might come in handy. Extra paper underwear, pads, soap, razor, numbing spray, and a plastic squirt bottle to help you rinse will probably be available so take advantage! You never know what may be useful to you at home. We also had to stop at the drug store on the way home because I had not yet prepared myself for delivery and did not have any pads, panty liners, over the counter pain reliever, or anything else recommended that would be necessary.

* * * * *

Make sure you take care of yourself. If you had a C-section remember to take the healing time you need. Your baby needs you healthy more than anything.

Tiny

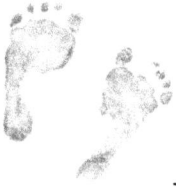

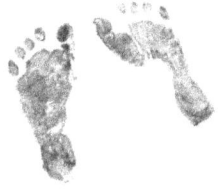

Being Discharged and Coming Home Without Baby

IT WAS PRETTY DEPRESSING TO COME HOME without my two babies. You see parents on T.V. bring their baby home to decorations and banners and signs and to friends and family who have come to meet the baby. We did not have that. We had not told anyone I had given birth except our parents, siblings, and best friends. It was too tenuous for us. Some people choose to let the world know when their baby has been born with an announcement and a photo, regardless of the gestational age, but we could not bring ourselves to send out those scary photos and let the world know the boys had arrived when there was a very real possibility that the one or both of the babies would not be coming home. We basically stopped posting on social media, did not call friends for a chat, and lived in a very small bubble for a very long time. When the boys were 6 weeks old I mentioned to one of the nurses that we had not told the world the boys had been born, and she was very supportive and acted like it was a logical choice. It was nice to feel that I was doing something right in a situation that was very wrong in every other way. She may have thought we were nuts because we waited that long without telling everyone, but one of the best things about NICU nurses is their ability to make you feel like you are parenting "right" regardless of what you are doing. Our homecoming was very bittersweet and nothing like I had pictured at all. It was quiet, somber, and involved a call to the NICU the minute we stepped into the door to begin our new life as parents.

The first thing I did when I got home was to take all my maternity clothing out of my closet. It made me unbelievably sad to look at it all hanging there, never to be worn. I had been lucky to receive hand-me-downs and bought myself a few new things, preparing for how big I was told I would get with twins. I had only gotten to wear a few things and now my pregnancy was over. Looking at the clothing made me feel sick and I wanted to cry. I should have still been pregnant. It was not fair. I felt like I had only recently gotten to the point where I looked obviously pregnant and not just overweight. I had had a total of 3 strangers smile at me and ask when I was due or if I knew what I was having. I had been so excited to be pregnant. I loved people asking. I loved wearing maternity clothing. I felt gypped. It was not fair. I should have been pregnant for FOUR more months. I should have had strangers gawk and be surprised that I was so big for only being so few months pregnant because I was pregnant with twins. I had looked forward to that. I wanted to be huge. I wanted to carry my boys for as long as I could and grow them as big as I could and be happy when my water broke and then give birth and be excited to call friends and family and let them know that our boys had arrived. I was not going to get any of that now. I wanted the clothes gone. I did not want to get dressed every morning and look at all that was not going to be.

I owned 4 pairs of yoga pants and 5 shirts that fit my (newly) enormous chest so I decided that was what I was going to wear until I fit into the rest of my clothing again. I was a solid 40 pounds over my pre-pregnancy weight, 10 pounds over even what I entered the hospital weighing (because of all the postpartum fluid retention and bags of I.V.). Only a handful of things I owned fit but I did not want to look at the maternity clothes, let alone wear any of them. I threw everything maternity, minus the few new shirts and leggings I had just bought for myself, into a big box and dropped it off at Goodwill®. I packed those new shirts and leggings into a box for a friend who was my size and pregnant and mailed it the next day. I saved one shirt. One special maternity shirt that I had only gotten to wear once, to remind me I had been pregnant with twins. Everything else needed to be out of my sight. I was mad and I was sad and I did not need one more reminder that I was not pregnant any longer. I even apologized at one point to the NICU nurses that they had to keep seeing me wear the same 5 shirts over and over because they were the only things that fit me. Of course they nicely said they had not noticed and did not care. They told me how great I looked and what mattered was that I was there with my babies who did not care what I was wearing.

The second thing I did the day I got home from the hospital was start the boys' calendars. I had received two 'My Life as a Baby' blank 12 month calendars at my baby shower from one of my best friend's moms. I started with the first blank month and filled in the days, beginning with the day each boy was born. I was now ready to record all their important events. The stickers that came with the calendars marked events like coming home, doctor visits, first words, first steps and usual things that happen in the first year of life. I knew we would not use those stickers for a long time, but it was helpful to start the calendars and record everything that was happening in the NICU so we would not forget anything.

* * * * *

There are first year preemie baby calendars available with stickers that record all the NICU events (vent, CPAP, bottle, clothes, I.V.s out, etc). We did not have those, but we wrote in our calendars a lot and used the stickers that came with them much later.

* * * * *

I also used the calendars to record everything from new foods to activities to fun outings. I ended up with another calendar for their second year to keep track of all their accomplishments and to finish using all the stickers.

THE THIRD THING I DID AT HOME WAS TO SET an alarm on my phone for every 3 hours for me to wake up and pump. I could not do much for the boys but I could do that. The NICU had sent me home with plastic containers for breastmilk and labels for each baby, and I was going to work my hardest to fill them up and bring them back every day.

* * * * *

For us, it was not helpful for friends and family to drop everything and rush to the hospital or our home after the boys were born. We did not have immediate family in the state and everyone's first inclination was to want to jump on a plane and physically be with us. Offering to do that was nice. It might have been helpful if we already had children who needed care while we were at the hospital. However, we had a plan for our dog (involving our neighbors, dog walker, and scheduling my NICU visits to allow for a midday trip home to let the dog out) and we did not have other children so having additional family members in our home would have been much harder to deal with than what they could have offered in terms of help. I was pumping every 3 hours around the clock in the living room and would not have wanted to have to move that whole set up to a private room to accommodate family members. For us, in those first NICU days and months, it made much more sense for our families to stay put until the boys were home.

* * * * *

It was difficult when we showed friends or family photos of our boys and the immediate response was "Oh, they're so small!" or "Wow, they're so much smaller than I thought they'd be". Preemie and micro preemie parents know how tiny our babies are. We are not proud of that. It is actually devastating. No one wants a tiny baby hooked up to machines. Everyone wants a nice big fat healthy baby. Reminding NICU parents how small or fragile looking their baby is probably does not feel good; they are thinking about that enough as it is. I would have much rather heard "I've never seen a 24 weeker, thank you for sharing that with me" or "I am thinking about you and hoping for good news soon". That is honest and straightforward. Also, parents cannot hear enough how beautiful their baby is. Every baby is beautiful, no matter how small or how many wires they have coming off them.

But Mighty

Tiny

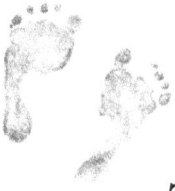

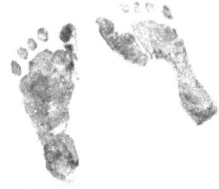

The New Normal of Life in the NICU

I CANNOT IMAGINE WANTING TO BECOME A neonatologist, a neonatal surgeon, a neonatal nurse practitioner, or a neonatal nurse, but I have now met people who have become all of these things. These have to be among the most emotionally draining, stressful, and detail oriented professions in the world. However, I am eternally grateful for anyone who chose these professions. Most every preemie and micro preemie parent says this, but I know that WE really had the best doctors, surgeons, nurse practitioners and nurses in the world. During one of our very first visits to the NICU, before I had even been discharged from the hospital, one of the nurses gave us a quick tour to show us where everything was. She showed us the Ronald McDonald House™ overnight rooms and kitchenette, told us how to put our name in for a room (they are like small very basic hotel rooms, assigned on a first come/first served basis, with priority given to parents with children having surgery), the washer and dryer, the pumping room where I was relieved to find I did not need to cart my newly rented heavy duty hospital grade pump back and forth to the hospital every day but instead could bring only the pumping parts I needed, and the bathroom. And she was so nice. They are all so nice, and caring, and there for you.

The first days, when I had a million questions and did not know anything about anything, the NICU nurses answered every question I had. They did it happily. They made me feel as though I was the first person who had ever asked that question and not as though it was the hundredth time that week that they had to explain the exact same thing. They made me feel like everything I was doing was okay and that our boys were well taken care of.

The boys did not start out in the same room in the NICU. They were on either side (A and B) of a large divided room (pod) because babies are placed in isolettes (incubators) or warming beds or cribs according to when they are born and the baby's needs. Even if my boys had been born at the same time and arrived at the NICU together, they would not have been placed in the same side of the pod because of the amount of care they each required. My boys were the only micro preemies in the pod. There were other preemies. There were also a few full term babies who had various issues that necessitated more care than the regular nursery provides.

At the time of their births, the boys were so needy that their NICU nurse only cared for one other healthier baby. It would have been too much for one nurse to care for both our boys at the same time. Everyone kept apologizing that the boys were on either side of the pod, but frankly walking back and forth between them during my visits gave me something more to do. During the first few days I was only allowed to touch the boys gently and with even pressure for minutes at a time. Too much touch would be too much of a stimulant and detrimental to them. Stroking them was too hard on their wet, thin, nearly translucent skin; therefore, for a long time we put one finger up against their foot to let them know we were there. During the first few days I spent with them, it was actually nice to sit and watch one, touch him for a few minutes and talk quietly to him, and then leave the room, use sanitizer, and do the same thing again on the other side of the pod to the other.

At first there was nothing to do but watch them and talk to them. I felt guilty when I was not there, but when I was there I felt useless. The first week I brought and wrote thank you notes for my baby shower gifts and I read a book in between touching and watching the boys. It was the only thing I could think to do to make my stay longer. The entire rest of the time I visited the NICU I never saw someone else do the same thing. If the nurses thought it was odd, they never let on. I felt like I needed to be there but while I was there I could not do anything. Other parents seemed to visit less frequently or for less time each day or had babies who were much older and bigger so parents could hold and play with them. I felt like I was the only one in my situation for a long time.

Phone calls needed to be made in the hall and not in the pod, so every morning when I arrived I would snap a few photos for my husband and then step into the hall to send them and call him with an update. I spent the first few days getting used to the constant dinging and beeping of the machines and monitors, the flashing lights, ventilator hum, the hustle and bustle and routine of the NICU. There is never a silent moment in the NICU. It takes some time to get used to the constant noise. It also takes some time, for someone outside the medical profession, to get used to the doctors and nurses reacting to the alarms. And there are lots of monitors and lots of alarms.

* * * * *

One of the first questions our friends and family asked initially and that we were asked again much later when we announced their births was how long our babies would need to be in the NICU. The truth was we did not know. Doctors and nurses try not to give discharge timeframes as much as possible because anything that can happen can change the course of a NICU stay and dramatically increase or decrease the time a baby needs care. Most typically, I have heard nurses estimate that around the baby's due date is usually a good ballpark date for discharge of a preemie. Micro preemies typically need more time than that. The boys were born at the end of April and we were told to think about spending the whole summer and hopefully not too much of the fall in NICU.

* * * * *

Different NICUs may have different rules about who can bring visitors back to see the baby. Married couples may both be allowed to visit the baby as well as bring back visitors, while unmarried couples may find only the biological mother is allowed to visit on her own and needs to be present for others to visit. This may complicate visiting times and may create a lot of pressure for the mother to be there in order for other friends and family to see the baby. It may be important to remember that mom is also trying to rest and recuperate from giving birth and too many visitors may be too much to handle right away.

* * * *

Family and friends might not be invited to visit with the babies in the NICU right away or at all. When the babies first arrived we were actually advised by our nurses that additional visitors could create more stress for the babies (more activity, louder voices, more commotion) and do more harm than good. Do not feel badly if you live in the area but are not asked to come and visit the baby in the NICU. There will be plenty of time for visiting once the baby comes home.

* * * *

During the first week we started posting to a website called Caring-Bridge. This non-profit organization allows you to write public or password protected blogs so that during a medical crisis or any personal challenge one person can post information and updates to keep multiple friends and family members all informed. This became a lifesaver. Initially we were fielding phone calls from a very small number of friends and family, but along the way, as the boys grew, that circle expanded. With CaringBridge I was able to post information every day and friends and family were able to log on at their leisure to get caught up on the boys' progress. That way, I did not have to relay the same information by text and phone call to everyone who cared how the boys were doing.

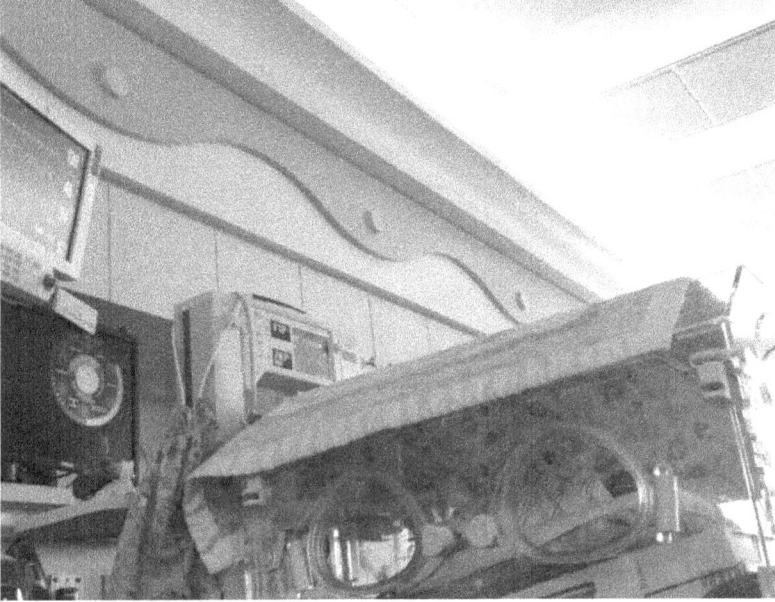

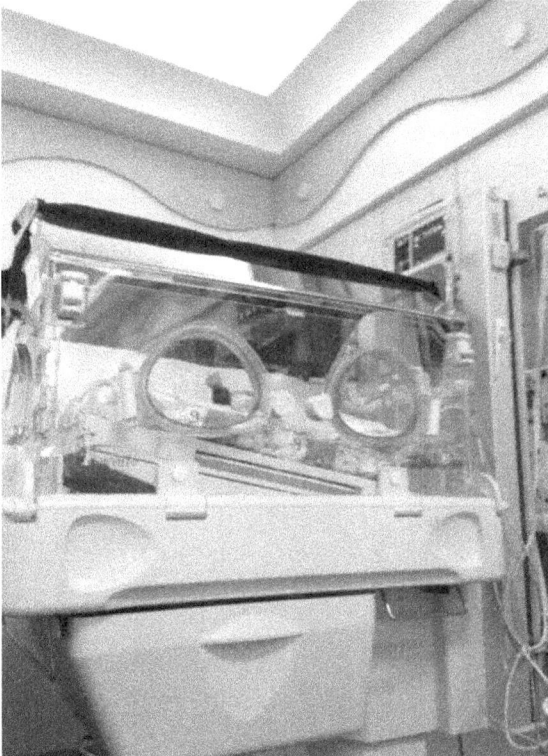

Tiny

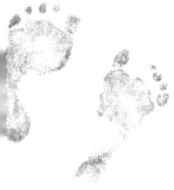

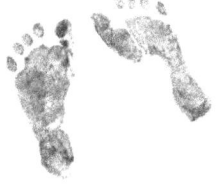

You May Cry a Lot…or Not at All

I HAVE HEARD PERSONAL STORIES OF MANY parents of premature babies about how much they cried when they first had their baby or when they were discharged from the hospital or every time they left the NICU without their baby or just randomly through the day during their journey. They have also told me they cried over happy milestones, such as when they got to hold their baby for the first time or when the baby was finally able to come home.

Dealing with emotions and hormones after giving birth to one or multiple babies is hard enough, but to put the additional stress and emotion of having a baby or babies in the NICU on top of that can be overwhelming. Crying, even at the drop of a hat, is totally understandable. That is what I would have expected for myself if I had known what our situation was going to be. However, I had the opposite reaction. I felt that if I started crying I would never stop. I felt as though I had to focus on what I could do for the boys. I did not want to stop to think about how sad I was or become emotional about their situation so I did not cry at all. It might not be what a psychologist would deem the healthiest way to deal with the boys' NICU time, but it was what worked for me. I felt like I had to be strong for the boys, which was how I dealt with the emotions.

There were certainly times, sometimes on the drive to the hospital when I would hear a poignant song on the radio, when I would feel as though I could have a complete breakdown and cry hysterically. But at those times I felt more compelled to tamp that down, swallow, and think about what I was going to do to help the boys when I got there. I would think about how I needed to be strong and get things done. I never had the moment when I felt like I broke and sobbed it all out. I might have needed to, or even benefited from having done so, but at the time it was not something I felt I could let myself do. I am not sure I would advise anyone that it was the best strategy for dealing with the sadness, anger, resentment, and devastation I felt, but at the time it was what felt good to me.

* * * * *

You may cry a lot, or not at all. Whatever truly helps you get through this time is what you should do.

* * * * *

I heard a lot during this time, as I am sure many others in situations like ours have, "I don't know how you do it." I understand the sentiment; it is very nice to have someone acknowledge that what you are going through seems hugely challenging and like an enormous burden and they think you are handling it well. However, I never really had a good response to being told "I don't know how you do it". In my mind I would think "You just do. If you had to, you'd just do it too". I was not doing anything special or out of the ordinary; I was simply doing what had to be done and what the doctors and nurses were telling me to do. Sure, it was a lot to handle. No, it was not easy. But we could always see how much luckier we were than others who were in much more dire situations than we were. It never proved to be a very good conversation starter when someone would tell me that. I think perhaps, "You're doing great" or "Keep it up" would have been more encouraging and helpful to hear.

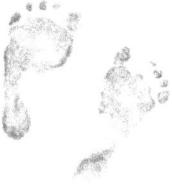

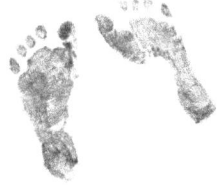

The Breast Pump: Your New Best Friend

I HAD NOT REGISTERED FOR OR PURCHASED a breast pump because I had my heart set on breastfeeding. I had planned to rent one from the hospital if the need arose, but I had hoped to only use one for a short time initially, if at all, to help put some milk in the freezer for occasional bottle feeds. When I told my OB/GYN during one of my initial routine visits that I planned on breastfeeding twins, he broke out his famous "It's good to have goals." He was right, obviously, because even the most fervent and heartfelt attempts at breastfeeding do not always go according to what mom would like. He told me that while that was a wonderful goal, he wanted to make sure I was not afraid of formula, pumping or turning to formula if we needed it to supplement or if something prevented me from being able to breastfeed. Since the boys were now obviously not going to be able to breastfeed initially, if ever, I needed to start pumping. Within hours of delivery I had my newly rented hospital breast pump and was briefly taught how to put the strange and foreign looking parts together and I began pumping.

For 10 minutes every hour, night and day, for the first few days, I pumped. Washing pumping parts in a tiny hospital recovery room sink was not ideal, but we made it work. I was lucky to begin producing colostrum almost immediately. I never felt my milk "come in," as I have heard it described by others. I did not wake up one morning and all of a sudden have a full supply, but I slowly began to produce more and more to deliver to the NICU. After I was discharged, I kept pumping at home and either freezing the milk or bringing it back to the NICU.

It was not until later on that I learned how important providing breastmilk to micro preemies is. Two of the most detrimental things micro preemies face are infections and Necrotizing Enterocolitis (NEC), the infection, death or perforation of some part of the intestinal tract. With micro preemies, formula fed babies are between 6 and 10 times more likely to face NEC than breastmilk fed babies and for older preemies (closer to 36 weeks) the risks are 20 times greater. Formula fed premature babies are also twice as likely to have systemic infections like sepsis as breast fed babies are. Breastmilk even cuts the risk for Retinopathy of Prematurity (ROP), an eye disease, in half. Breastmilk fed preemies and micro preemies are shown in study after study to do better and leave the hospital sooner when compared with formula fed babies. At the time I did not realize it, but I was not only doing the only thing I could for the boys I was actually increasing their chances of surviving and thriving while doing it.

Having a baby or babies in the NICU is unbelievably stressful. My husband served in the military and spent 12 months at war in Iraq. I certainly do not know what the experience was like for him, but I know how stressful it was for me. Having my boys in the NICU was far more stressful. Stress is one of the main reasons women who would like to be breastfeeding or pumping are not able to do so. I was very lucky that pumping was not something I was having a hard time with and was something I felt positive about doing for my babies.

* * * * *

In cases where mom is not able to provide breastmilk some hospitals offer donor breastmilk as a substitute. In other hospitals donor milk can be requested and in still others it can be purchased. If you are not able to provide breastmilk, you can talk to your NICU neonatologist and NICU nurses about the ways in which your baby can receive breastmilk.

IN ADDITION TO VISITING WITH THE BOYS, I did a lot of eating and a lot of pumping while I was at the hospital. After the first few days I was pumping for 25 minutes every 3 hours, around the clock, as instructed by the lactation consultant at the hospital. Pumping now dictated basically my entire day. I had my phone alarm set to go off every 3 hours to remind me to pump. I began planning when I would leave the house for the hospital, when I would leave the hospital for home, and basically when I did anything around when I had to pump next. I usually pumped immediately before I left for the hospital, so that after the long drive to get there I still had a little time to visit with the boys before I had to pump again. I tried to pump right before I left the hospital to allow me time to get something done on the way home or at home before I had to stop and pump again. Pumping dictated when I left the house again to get my husband after he finished work on the way to the hospital for the second visit of the day, and it dictated when I left him alone to visit with the boys while I pumped before we went home. And on and on.

For me, the feeling the breast pump provided varied from almost unnoticeable to incredibly painful. Somehow I initially missed the memo on using some kind of lubricant in the flanges while pumping so that it did not feel as though the pump was basically trying to rip my breasts from my body. Because of that, the first few lubricant-less weeks were tough. When I was finally found the miracle product that is Lanolin, the game changed. Pumping was not excruciating anymore. For the majority of the time I pumped, it was just uncomfortable.

Months later, when I experimented with a different set of flanges, it became even less uncomfortable. The new flanges also gave me an 'empty' feeling for the first time and increased how much milk I was able to pump. But it always had an ever-present not great feeling. There is not a lot of time between setting up to pump, pumping for 25 minutes, cleaning all the pump parts for a few minutes, putting the milk into storage containers and labeling them properly before then having to begin it all again. I was basically left with 2 hours with which to visit-if I was at the hospital, sleep-if it was the middle of the night, drive-if I was on my way to the hospital or home from it, or if I was home-walk the dog/feed the dog/clean the house/write thank you notes/grocery shop/iron/do laundry/eat/do errands/talk on the phone/ call the NICU/take a shower/fold laundry/make dinner/make lunch/ make breakfast/pack my bag for the hospital/everything else it takes to live. Two hours is not a lot of time. Everyone kept telling me to take a nap or take it easy. There just was not a lot of time for that.

I would usually use the time while I was pumping, since I started using a hands-free double pumping bra from day 1, to text an update to someone, post an update on CaringBridge, or eat. I ate a lot. Pumping for twins can require almost 500 extra calories a day. I got hungry in the middle of the night so I started stocking the house and my nightstand with protein bars. It was helpful to have something I could grab in the dark and eat quickly and easily to help me go right back to sleep. While I was at the NICU I usually ate my lunch in the pumping room to save the time of having to leave the boys and eat it in the Ronald McDonald House™ lounge. Peanut butter and jelly sandwiches became my almost daily lunch because they were easy to eat with one hand, quiet, and calorically dense. They say breastfeeding is one of the best ways to lose pregnancy weight. I cannot speak to breastfeeding since pumping can be different, but I did lose about 4 pounds a day for almost the first two weeks while eating everything in sight plus a pint of Ben & Jerry's every night. The ice cream was the best part of those first two weeks.

* * * * *

Start pumping immediately – it is literally the best thing you can be doing for your baby and the one thing no one else can do.

* * * * *

Use the lactation specialists at the hospital; they have a wealth of knowledge and are there to help you. Kellymom is another online resource for all things pumping and breastfeeding. Moms groups or breastfeeding support groups in person or online are also great resources. Chances are someone has been in your shoes and can answer questions you may have. The lactation consultants can probably direct you to a breastfeeding support groups also.

* * * * *

If you do not own a breast pump, rent a hospital grade pump from the hospital. They are designed to be the most efficient, and efficiency is key when pumping for a baby in the NICU and for pumping later on if you are trying to supply for multiples.

* * * * *

Use Lanolin or another oil-based lubricant in the flanges every time you pump.

* * * * *

Try different flanges if you think you are not getting a good fit or if you are uncomfortable. Heck, try others even if you think you are comfortable. I did not know what I was missing until I tried the Pumpin' Pals Super Shields™. I do not receive any compensation for pushing their product but I recommend it to every new mother I know. Immediately my supply went up and I realized what it was like to feel empty when I started using them. You may not know what you are missing unless you try something different.

* * * * *

Try various nursing pads. The kind I liked better than the washable cotton pads I began with were called Lilypadz® and were made of thin flexible silicone. Because the silicone did not absorb the Lanolin like the cotton pads did, I could reapply it a few times a day rather than every time I pumped. Make sure you are washing well to get all the Lanolin off and letting your breasts dry well every day so that your skin stays healthy.

* * * * *

Make sure you pay attention to your body. If something feels physically off, say something to a nurse or your OB/GYN. You cannot visit your baby if you are sick.

* * * * *

I started carrying my pumping parts to and from the hospital in a gallon sized zip top bag, but they did not have the time or opportunity to dry between pumping and cleaning that way. My aunt graciously sewed me some cotton Velcro topped bags the same size and they worked much better at allowing the parts to dry completely because they allowed air to circulate.

* * * * *

Pack an extra bottle brush and small bottle of dish detergent in a zip top bag to take to the hospital. The NICU pumping area would sometimes run out of detergent with which to wash my pumping containers and parts.

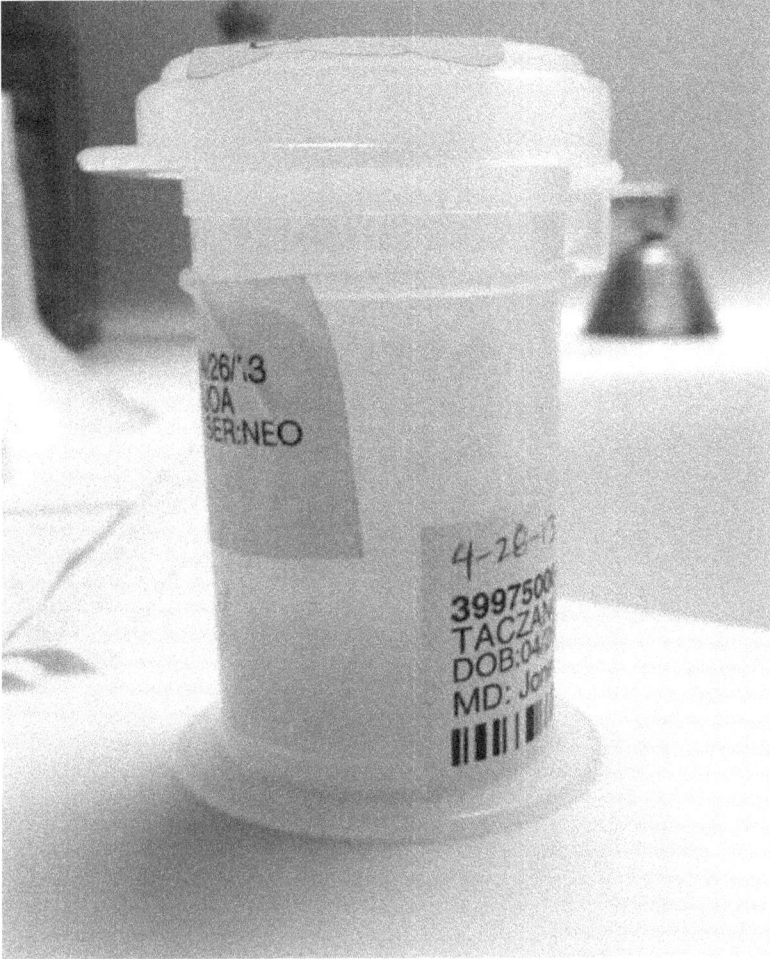

Tiny

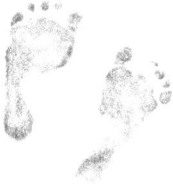

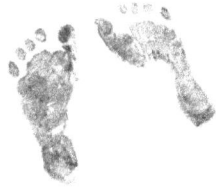

The NICU

AT FIRST, I FELT THE BOYS WERE HOOKED UP to just about every machine the NICU had to offer. Although Chuck started out on the CPAP, he got tired after a few hours and could not breathe on his own and was intubated and put on a ventilator. Henry was intubated at birth and so began life on a ventilator. These machines were doing all the breathing work for the boys by forcing warm moist air into their lungs because they were not old or strong enough to breathe by themselves. The vents were programed to give a certain number of breaths per minute, to have a certain length to each breath, and to allow for additional oxygen to be given with each breath.

Babies born prematurely are now monitored very closely to only receive the minimum amount of additional oxygen possible. Too much oxygen can lead to ROP. ROP was responsible for the visual problems and blindness in very premature babies in much larger numbers in the past than it is today, thanks to the close monitoring and early interventions to treat ROP. The boys had leads on their stomachs to monitor their heartbeat and breaths, oxygen saturation monitors (Pulse Ox) wrapped around their feet, UV lights above them to fight off jaundice from too high a concentration of bilirubin, and blood pressure cuffs on their legs. At birth they had intravenous lines inserted into their umbilical cords. They both had Orogastric Tubes (OT tube) that went into their mouths and all the way into their bellies. They had lots of wires coming off them. Because of the ventilators and the masks to shield their eye from the lights, we could not see much of their faces. Their eyelids had not yet developed enough to physically open (that happens later on in the womb) so they were still fused shut. Their diapers, so small they fit in the palm of my hand, were so large on them they covered some of their stomach and most of their thighs. Because their skin had not completed development yet it was tacky and sticky to the touch and almost translucent looking. Their incubators were humidified and heated so they were warm and moist and had two holes into which the nurses could put their hands to work on the baby. They lay on a moldable pillow (Z-Flo®) to cradle their body and allow their position to be changed every few hours to be kept as comfortable as possible. It took some time to get used to seeing our babies like that. It was pretty scary.

It also took some time to get used to the routine of the NICU. Although, as parents, we were allowed to visit 22 hours of the day, we were prohibited for an hour during the nurses' shift change at 7 am and 7 pm every day. We were allowed to bring in a certain number of visitors during the rest of the time as well, except for during rounds when the neonatologist attending physician, neonatologist fellow, nurse practitioner, and other staff rounded on each baby to go over how that baby had done during the previous 24 hours and outline a game plan for the next 24 hours. During this time only parents were allowed in the pod. Because the boys were in the NICU of a teaching hospital, our neonatologist attending physician rotated monthly. I always thought that was to our advantage since it allowed for new eyes and perhaps new ideas. I felt we always benefited from changes made when attending physicians rotated.

* * * * *

You can call the NICU 24 hours a day, 7 days a week to get an update on your baby. You may not always reach your baby's nurse at that moment (this happens every so often) because they may be in the middle of dealing with another baby, but you can call back or they can call you back. You are not annoying them. They do not want you to worry and they want you to know how your baby is doing.

* * * * *

Not every phone call from the NICU is bad news. To be honest, the majority of phone calls probably will not be great news. Doctors, nurse practitioners and nurses are ridiculously busy and if they get to know your visiting schedule and know you will be in that day, they will probably save good news for when they see you or they will pass it on to the next nurse who will see you. But try not to have your heart in your throat and immediately panic when you see the phone number. We received more than one phone call with great news. Most likely, even when the phone call is not positive, the immediate problem has already been resolved and someone is just calling to let you know what actions have been taken. Nurses will address whatever problem arises and then call you; they do not stop in the middle. So whatever crisis they are informing you of has likely passed. Therefore, panicking and driving 90 miles an hour back to the hospital is not in yours or your baby's best interest.

* * * * *

Write down the name of your attending, fellow, nurse practitioner, and nurse. You can ask to speak with them after rounds if you need to. Attendings and fellows are in charge of lots of babies, so they are not always at your immediate disposal, but try their hardest to speak with you individually during rounds or throughout the day if you can let your baby's nurse know.

* * * * *

Write down your baby's vital signs and monitor settings as you get to know them to see how they vary day to day. You will get a better idea of your baby's "normal" that way. Certainly the nurses will know from pervious notes what has improved or not for your baby, but no one should know your baby better than you. I always wrote down the boys' vent settings before I left so I would know when I called later that day or that night if they had changed and I could compare and know if things had improved or declined. I also got to know their typical heart rate and blood pressure (which were very different from each other) so that if there was a new nurse I could give them an idea of what seemed off or not.

* * * * *

Wear layers to the hospital in case you get hot or cold. Most days I ended up wearing stretch pants and a t-shirt with a long sleeved hooded sweatshirt, sneakers and socks. It felt weird for a very long time to wear open toed shoes because I felt like it was not clean enough. Hospitals are typically cold and the NICU is not much of an exception. The doctors and nurses who work there all day are running around-sometimes literally running- so the temperature always felt cool while I just sat and I needed the long sleeves and long pants. I was also pumping every 3 hours around the clock, so it was easy to take off a sweatshirt and lift up a t-shirt to pump as opposed to wearing something more bulky.

* * * * *

Bring hand cream in case your hands get dry from the extreme washing and sanitizing.

* * * * *

Bring something to take notes with (paper/pen, phone) because you will probably think of things you need to do at home or want to bring with you while you are there.

* * * * *

Bring in things from home. It may feel weird but having your baby lying on their own blanket from home, taping a photo in their incubator or putting up a family picture is important. You are responsible for washing linen brought from home. Label blankets to ensure they do not get confused with hospital linen. I tried permanent marker, but it actually began to wash out and become illegible. Instead, I ordered embroidered laundry tags with our last name and I sewed them on every blanket, swaddle wrap, and quilt we brought in (not clothing). Linens are changed daily, if not more often (when medication, blood, or anything else gets spilled on them) in the incubators, so you may go through a lot of blankets. Your nurse may have somewhere for you to store extras.

*****

Hydrogen peroxide is great at getting blood or other bodily fluids out of blankets or clothing before washing.

* * * * *

We were very lucky to have friends and family who could not wait to be told what they could do to help us. But, frankly, there was not a whole lot in the beginning for them to do as we were trying to simply get through each day. Some things, however, were unbelievably nice to have done for us. Think about what else NICU parents have to take care of besides visiting with their baby and perhaps offer to take something off their plate. My husband's company was extremely supportive and began paying to have a yard service do our mowing and edging. They did this for 6 months to allow us time to focus on the boys and ourselves. Whether yard work, childcare for siblings, grocery shopping or anything that takes attention away from a baby in the hospital, offer to help with that. We were also gifted a home cleaning visit by a cousin which was wonderful. Eventually, when we were able to clothe and swaddle the boys, we had cousins who were happy to provide those items, which can be expensive if they are special preemie or micro preemie sizes.

* * * * *

Providing meals is a wonderful thing. My husband's company took turns providing us a meal every Friday for months. It was such a relief to know we had something fresh to eat Friday when we got home from our late NICU visit and also for the next few lunches and dinners as well. Having a meal delivered is also appreciated. Whether it was a neighbor bringing over a casserole or a cousin contacting our favorite restaurant and arranging dinner for 4 to be delivered every Tuesday for months, it all takes a little something off the plate of a NICU parent. Those meals went a long way and we looked forward to them. My brother and a friend both called in pizza delivery so all we had to do was open the door and dinner was ready. All of that was much appreciated.

* * * * *

We ended up eating a lot of sandwiches. I needed to eat breakfast on my way to the NICU every morning, needed a lunch while I was there, and picked up my husband to drive back every evening. Sandwiches were the easiest thing for us to eat in the car. We were given a whole spiral ham, loaves of bread and individual bags of chips by my husband's boss, so I had ham sandwiches for breakfast, lunch and dinner for 2 weeks straight. I was tired from pumping, stressed from the entire situation, and just trying to make it to the next day so I did not care what I was eating; it was just nice when it was planned for me, easy and filling.

* * * * *

We received gift cards for easy take-out at restaurants located close to the hospital and around home. Those meals were a highlight also.

ALL OF THE LIGHTS AND WIRES AND SOUNDS of the NICU are hard to get used to at first. Sometimes the room felt very full of people and I felt as though I was in the way. It did not matter how many times the nurse would warmly offer me a chair for me to sit on to see into the incubator (which was raised to arm height for the nurses to easily reach in to care for the boys but hard to see into from anything but a high chair), I still felt as though I was invading their space and getting in their way. During the first few rounds I listened to the doctors and nurses talk about the babies that I, as their mother, was supposed to be caring for and yet could not. I was unable to offer anything productive, let alone understand half of what was said. I spent a lot of time writing down things I did not understand to ask a nurse later. As the days passed, I was able to follow the conversation more closely and understand what was being discussed. After rounds I would step into the hall and text my husband with an update. Initially there was a lot of watching and looking and not a lot of being able to do much.

Even though it did not feel like much, I could actually help do some things for our tiny babies from day one. Help might be a strong word, since obviously the nurses were much faster and incalculably better at doing these things, but my husband and I were able to do them nonetheless and it made us feel as though we were a part of the boys' care. It was hard to not be scared that when I touched one of the boys I was not going to screw something up, like disconnect a wire and have something catastrophic happen. They were so tiny and they had so many wires coming off of them. The vent tube was also very finicky and could not be moved very much, which is why the boys were handled slowly, delicately and really only when necessary.

Our nurses were very specific and informative about what we could touch, what we should avoid touching, and what we could do for the boys. It was helpful to get in there early and overcome the fear of breaking them. Before Henry was a week old, we had both changed his diaper. That may not seem like much to most parents, but for us it was a huge milestone. I was even able to pick up his tiny body and hold him with two hands while his nurse changed a blanket underneath him. It was very difficult for me, especially after seeing the way the nurses are able to both hold the baby and the vent tube and change the blanket quickly and practically one handed. I, on the other, needed both hands to make sure I was holding him correctly and could not do anything else. Every 3 hours the nurse would have to take a blood pressure, temperature, and other vital signs and reposition the baby slightly. When we were present, we were allowed to do those things also. The nurses tried to include us and made it feel like a big deal even when we were doing the same things they had done thousands of times before. Within the first few weeks we were able to help with sponge baths, taking vitals, feeding with syringes into the OG tube, and holding pacifiers.

* * * * *

Do not be shy about asking what you can help with and what you can be a part of. By the end of our stay, one of the techs mistook me for a new nurse practitioner as I took care of my son. The nurses and I all laughed, but you will be surprised what you will get used to and become good at. The worst a nurse or doctor can say is that you cannot help with something, and no one will be angry with you for asking. Even though the nurses listened to the boys' hearts and bellies every 3 hours, it was months before someone offered for me to listen to their hearts. It simply had not occurred to me to ask.

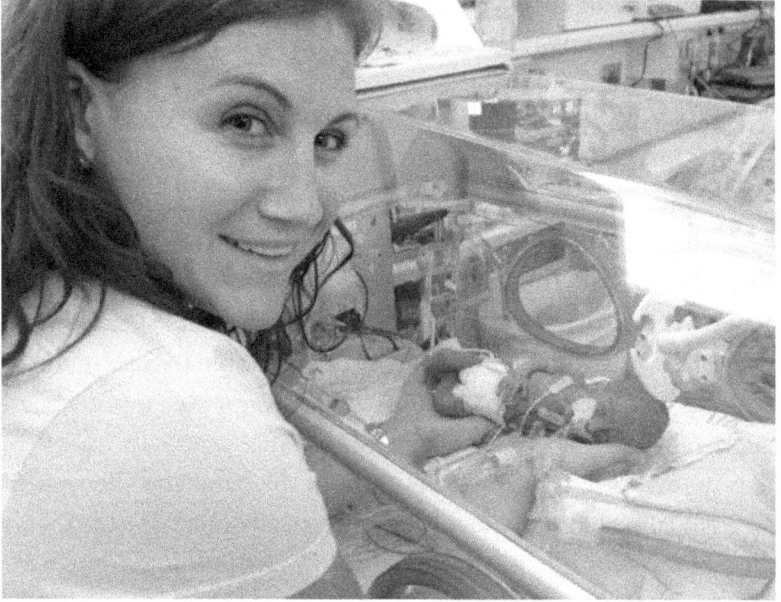

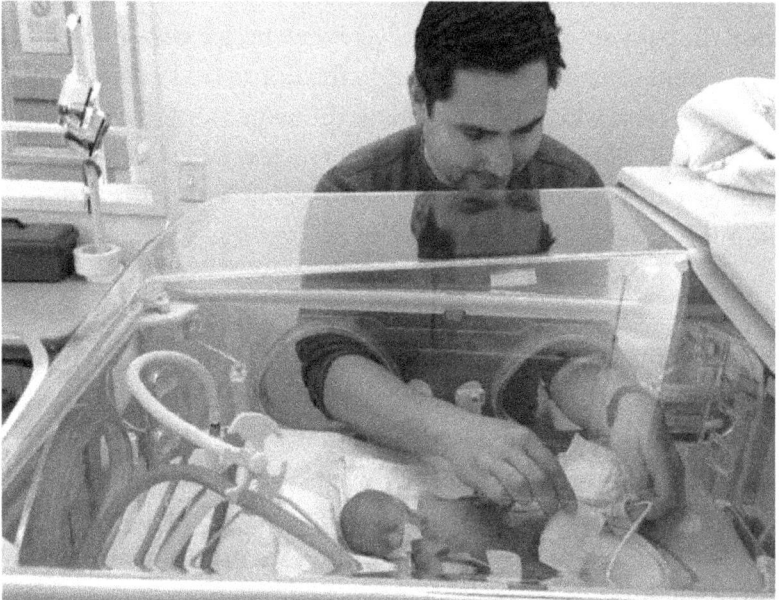

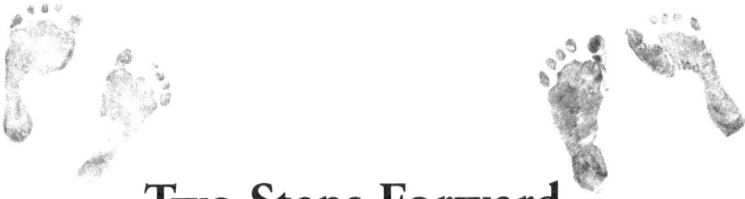

Two Steps Forward and One Step Back

AS DAYS TURNED INTO WEEKS WE CELEBRATED the smallest victories the boys accomplished. Their first poop (poop is a big deal in the NICU), first feeding (1 cc of breastmilk, given by syringe into the OG tube directly into the belly), first time they opened their eyes once they were off the bili lights. All those things were important steps in the right direction. Lots of things can go wrong very quickly with mirco preemies and preemies, but lots of things can go amazingly right also. One of our nurses told us life in the NICU is like a roller-coaster, uphill and downhill, two steps forward and one step back. That definitely proved to be correct for us. It is wonderful when a baby has a short NICU stay with no setbacks, but babies born very prematurely who experience that are more the exception than the rule. It is wonderful to celebrate your baby's victories, but I always tried to be cognizant of those around me who may not be celebrating that day.

For their first 3 days the boys did better than was expected. Unfortunately not many babies born as early as ours sail through all their NICU days. We had a major setback after those first few days. Chuck had a fairly common complication micro preemies can have, a perforated bowel. Nectorizing Entercolitis can cause bowel death and perforations in micro preemies, but Chuck was lucky that he did not have that along with the bowel perforation. NEC affects up to 12% of micro preemies and is fatal 30% of the time. At the time I did not realize it, because pumping or breastfeeding had always been my plan, but giving micro preemies breastmilk is a major factor in lessening the risk for NEC and also for reducing likelihood of bowel perforations. Luckily I was able to provide a never ending supply of breastmilk to the NICU for the boys, but this was not able to stave off the tiny hole in Chuck's very premature bowel. In Chuck's case, I noticed his belly looked swollen (his whole body was, in fact, very swollen and purple and bruised in places from the 'trauma' of birth) and mentioned it to his nurse. She paid attention and watched him and passed the information on to his next nurse, who noticed it worsening and alerted the fellow, who ordered an x-ray which showed air in his intestine and indicated a probable perforation in his bowel.

It was only the morning of my second day home after discharge and I was getting ready to make the trek to the hospital when we got the phone call from the pediatric surgery (Pedi Surg) team letting us know they had diagnosed Chuck's problem and needed us to come to the hospital immediately to discuss the next course of action. Of course it was heart stopping. The surgeon even had to ask me how long it would take us to get to the hospital to know whether or not they could wait to speak with us or if they would have to speak with us over the phone before proceeding. When someone asks you how long it is going to take you to drive to the hospital, you know how very serious the problem is. I immediately raced to my husband's office, we drove down and we ran from the parking garage and were standing in the NICU within 50 minutes.

When we spoke with the surgical attending and fellow, we were faced with a difficult decision. For the type of problem Chuck had, there is not consensus among neonatal surgeons as to the best course of treatment. A minor surgery can be performed wherein a drain is inserted into the abdomen with the hope that the intestine only has a very small perforation, minimal infection, and can repair itself without worsening (antibiotics would also be prescribed). Alternatively, a much larger and more invasive surgery can be performed wherein an incision is made in the baby's belly, the intestine pulled out and 'run' (the surgeon goes over every inch trying to find holes or infection) and the perforation and/or dead intestine is removed (and antibiotics are given). The healthy ends of intestine are then brought through the skin of the baby's belly (a stoma) to allow the intestinal tract to heal and grow. Babies who have this surgery will have an ostomy and bag attached to their belly to collect their solid waste (poop). At some point when the baby is bigger and healthier (in most, not all cases) a reversal surgery is performed where the ends of the intestines are sewed back together, put back in the abdominal cavity, and the baby's belly sewn up.

Our surgeon made a very convincing case for either surgery. It is unbelievably difficult to be faced with making a decision as to which kind of surgery you are going to approve for your tiny baby when no one can tell you which will be better, which will be more successful, or even which they would want to do on their own child. For us, there was also a third option. There was, at that time, a nationwide study with the goal of determining which of these two kinds of surgeries is more successful so that one over the other could be recommended in the future. Because of his type of problem Chuck qualified for the study. If we opted to enroll him in the study, it would be the study that randomly assigned him to one of the two types of surgeries the Pedi Surg team would perform. The surgeons left my husband and me 5 minutes to make a decision. On one hand, we reasoned, it is almost as if his body had not realized he was sick. He did not have a fever, he was not showing increased oxygen requirement or anything that would indicate that he was having a problem, so doing the less invasive surgery would spare him major surgery and hopefully allow his body to heal itself. It was an optimal time for that less invasive surgery. However, if it did not work, the more major surgery could be required. By that point, one would assume, Chuck would be feeling sicker and his body would be less likely to come through the more major surgery as easily. On the other hand, he was not feeling sick and his body was doing well so if we went ahead and opted for the major surgery now he would possibly have a better outcome from it than if he had to have it later.

After a few minutes of back and forth what we decided was that we could not make a decision. Both options had as many pros as cons and there was not a good way for us to make the decision for either surgery. Therefore, we opted to enroll him in the study. Immediately, cordless phone in hand, the surgical fellow called the study phone number and in moments he was enrolled and randomly assigned to have the more invasive surgery. After that decision was made, we had to wait for his turn for surgery behind one of his podmates. In the hour and a half since we had gotten the first phone call another baby had presented with NEC, only that baby was much sicker and required surgery first. It was reassuring to know our baby was stable enough to wait for surgery and heartbreaking to know another was not.

In the NICU, when babies are not stable enough to risk transportation to the surgical suites on another floor Pedi Surg, in essence, brings the surgical suite to the baby. The pediatric anesthesiologist and surgical team closes the baby's pod to all visitors (even parents of other babies) and lifts the lid off the baby's incubator to perform surgery right there where they have been laying. Through a sliver of the window of the door we could actually watch the surgery being performed. I chose to spend the hour the surgery took sitting by Henry and repeating over and over again silently "He's going to be okay". It was the longest hour of my life.

The relief when the surgeon popped his head in the doorway to tell me everything had gone as well as they could have hoped was immense. He said the next 24-48 hours would be critical, but he was optimistic. Henry's nurse was waiting for news also and she hugged me. We were lucky that Chuck had the best case scenario of a very serious diagnosis. He only had 1 tiny perforation, with no dead intestine, so only 2 cm of bowel had to be removed. For a scenario as serious as Chuck's, that is about as good as it gets. He made it through surgery and we celebrated his success. We were in such a panic we had not thought to drive to the hospital in two cars, but I now wanted to stay overnight to be close in case anything changed. We, therefore, drove home together, I packed a bag, and I drove back to stay the night in the Ronald McDonald House™ room. While Chuck was having surgery, one of the NICU nurses had called and reserved me a room in case I wanted it.

* * * * *

Many children's hospitals have Ronald McDonald House™ rooms either in the hospital itself or nearby. They are free to parents and available on a first come/first served basis. We were lucky that we lived only 45 minutes from the hospital so I was able to visit twice a day.

Even still, we utilized the Ronald McDonald House™ twice and were extremely glad it was there. Your baby's nurse can help you put your name on the list for a room if you need one. If one is not available, you can stay at baby's bedside 23 hours a day including overnight. Usually there are comfortable reclining chairs for parents to stay overnight next to baby if need be. It is not common but it is allowed.

* * * * *

It is wonderful to know friends and family care about you and are thinking about you. It is not helpful to leave many messages and ask that they be returned, especially in the middle of a crisis or setback. Parents are unbelievably stressed, sleep deprived, and just trying to cope with this unexpected journey. Making sure friends and family know you are not expecting a phone call in return is helpful.

* * * * *

Asking specific questions about how tests have gone can be stressful for parents. If results are good, parents will probably be happy to let everyone know as soon as they can. If they are not, parents may need time to process new information before sharing it. We shared certain things relating to the boys' prognosis for long term growth and development with close friends and family that I chose not to post on CaringBridge.

DURING THE NEXT 6 DAYS THE BOYS IMPROVED, but the success of Chuck's surgery was short lived. During our night visit on day 6 after surgery, he squirmed so much during a diaper change that he opened his ostomy incision and some of his intestines started coming out. My husband was watching the nurse while I was in with Henry and literally watched it happen. At first we were more confused than panicked and hopeful that everything could be tucked back in somehow. However, when Pedi Surg came to take a look a few minutes later they realized it would require another immediate surgery to correct. Our 3 hour evening visit after work turned into a 6 hour visit while we waited for Chuck to have surgery for the second time. Once surgery was finished and he was stable for a few hours, we finally drove home feeling drained.

Even without surgeries, preemies and micro preemies experience a lot of medications and changes. Initially, the boys' I.V. lines went directly through their umbilical cord. Those lines have a certain lifespan and cannot stay in place indefinitely. Within about a week a peripherally inserted central catheter (PICC) line had to be put in for the umbilical lines to be removed. Usually a PICC line is located on an arm and actually travels through the blood vessel up the arm towards the shoulder and ends close to the heart. Both boys had theirs placed at night by the line team because that is when the NICU is quietest and seems to work well for those procedures. The good thing about the PICC line was that it allowed for medications to be given without the baby needing to be stuck with a needle every time. It was also the line into which the total parenteral nutrition (TPN) was given, which helped keep the babies alive before they could get all their calories and nutrition from breastmilk.

* * * * *

Breastmilk is the clear winner when it comes to preemies and micro preemies. But if they cannot have that, for whatever reason, TPN is what supplies all they need to keep them growing. Remaining on TPN for prolonged periods of time has significant drawbacks; therefore, the goal was always to get back to breastmilk as soon as possible. The drawback to having a PICC line was that it was another opportunity for infection to enter and spread. It was a necessary evil that the boys needed until they could be trusted to remain stable and no longer need TPN. The PICC line was for things going in, but our boys also needed blood drawn out. Initially they would get heel pricks to draw blood to measure various things, mainly their blood gas. Their gasses determined their vent settings. If the boys were able to expel CO_2 properly, their vent settings decreased. If not, they were usually given more time and/or had their vent settings increased.

WE CALLED A LOT INITIALLY WHEN THE BOYS were getting gasses every 3 hours to ask what the latest numbers were. It was great news when they had a good number and were weaned on their vent and it was disappointing when they had to go up on their settings. They started out with the vents breathing entirely for them. We were told that they would have a certain time period to try to get off the vent without the help of steroids, but after a certain number of weeks the risks of the steroids would outweigh the risks of staying on the vents longer. The goal was to get off the vent as quickly as possible. It was by no means unusual that they needed the vent from birth, given how underdeveloped their lungs were. However, the less time they spent on the vents the better. The constant warm moist air being pumped into their lungs was a great environment for growing bacteria. Their blood, therefore, was cultured for a complete blood count (CBC) test multiple times a week at first, and then weekly as they grew, in order to be sure nothing looked abnormal. The CBC helped determine if there was any infection. Also, longer time spent on a vent can be associated with increased risks for Cerebral Palsy in babies.

The boys also received multiple head ultrasounds to look for any bleeding, or interventricular hemorrhages (IVH). IVHs are one of the common concerns with micro preemies because their blood vessels are so small and delicate they are easily torn during birth or shortly afterwards. IVHs are graded from 1-4, depending on severity, and can vary in how they may affect the baby long term. They can cause absolutely no damage in terms of development and motor skills, they can cause developmental delays that can be overcome with work and therapy, and they can also cause developmental problems that cannot be overcome. Ideally, a baby would have no bleeds, as was the case with Henry. Chuck, unfortunately, had a bleed on his first head ultrasound but it was not in the front top part of the brain where they are most commonly seen. His was in the cerebellum region at the back of his head and bleeds in that location are not graded. Since bleeds in that part of the brain are much less common, there was not as much information for us as to what this would mean for him. The best case scenario after seeing the bleed was that future ultrasounds would show first that it was not getting worse and second that it was being reabsorbed. Because their kidneys were so underdeveloped, both boys were on medications to help with urine output.

Also very commonly seen in micro preemies is a heart problem called Patent Ductus Arteriosus (PDA). In utero, the path the blood travels in the fetus bypasses the lungs, since they are not oxygenated and used to breathe air. This path changes at birth when the baby takes a first big breath. The big breath signals to the body to close the valve and change the path of the blood to include the lungs. The boys did not take a big breath so there was no signal to their heart to close the PDA and change the path of the blood. This valve remained open and caused the blood to flow throughout their body, predominantly bypassing the lungs and in doing so not picking up oxygen. This can be a contributing factor to mirco preemies having trouble supporting themselves without the vent. They need the extra support and oxygen from the vent because their own bodies are not functioning as they were intended to. Sometimes the PDA will close on its own, sometimes medication can be given that may close the PDA, and sometimes surgery is necessary.

Luckily, Chuck's PDA did not appear to be making him any worse and it was not significantly contributing to him needing extra vent support. That was a good thing because after his two surgeries he was not in a position to be given the medication or to have the surgery. The medication is only given up to a certain number of weeks after a baby is born, and Chuck was too sick within that window to receive it. For the time being, it was safer to watch his PDA and hope it closed on its own and he did not need surgery. Henry, on the other hand, had more trouble with his vent settings and his fellow believed the PDA was contributing to that. He received two rounds of the medication and that seemed to help shrink, but not close, the PDA. His vent settings after the medication were slightly improved so he would continue to work to get off the vent without surgery and the hope was his PDA would continue to close on its own. Nearly all babies with PDAs that are not closed with either surgery or medication will have a closed PDA by the time they are a few years old. As long as it was not showing signs of affecting anything else, Henry could live with it as it was.

* * * * *

Be conscious that babies are in the NICU for a large variety of reasons, but none of them are good. Your baby may be having a horrible day but someone else's could be going home. Sometimes that can lift your spirits and may help you to see that there is a light at the end of the tunnel. Alternatively, your baby may be having their best day but just a few incubators over someone else's suddenly crashes. The reality is not all babies are able to leave the NICU and go home. Remind your visitors to be quiet and discreet, even when celebrating your baby's achievement.

* * * * *

We were told stories from other preemie moms or from our friends and family about babies who had a medication one of our boys was going to be given or had a surgery that was a possibility for one of our boys. It was helpful to know that certain medications or procedures had been successful for other babies, but if then the medication did not work or the doctor decided the surgery was not a good idea, it was hard to switch gears in our heads. Lots of times we would be fearful and hope a surgery or medication would not be necessary, but then would hear how it had dramatically helped someone else's baby. We then began to think it could be a positive thing and got ourselves ready for it only to have something change and one of the boys not get whatever it was after all. Those changes in mindset were hard to keep going through. We just remained confident in our doctors and nurses that what worked for someone else's baby was not necessarily the best thing for ours.

BECAUSE OF HOW FRAGILE THE BOYS WERE and how sensitive their vents were to being moved and bumped it was exactly a month before we were allowed to hold them. Most of our friends and family had not thought about that. Lots of friends and family assumed we could begin holding our babies from their first day in the NICU, but that is not always the case with NICU babies. Although the NICU is extremely supportive and strongly encourages holding your infant skin-to-skin (kangaroo care), the baby has to meet certain criteria and be stable enough to do so. Once the baby is eligible, you have to be ready to hold the baby for at least a few hours. Otherwise, taking the baby out of their incubator, letting them get comfortable on your chest, and then putting them back in can be so stressful that it negates the benefits they receive from being held. After 4 weeks the boys were finally stable enough to be held and from that point we were able to hold them each once a day for a few hours.

* * * * *

For friends and family who have never seen a preemie or a micro preemie, the baby may look very different than you would picture. Rather than assuming parents are able to do a lot of things for the baby (such as holding them and feeding them), ask what they are able to do when they visit the NICU. It can be helpful for parents to feel like the severity of their situation is really understood.

* * * * *

Remember to eat, drink, go to the bathroom and pump before you kangaroo care. Nothing is worse than being in the middle of holding your baby and realizing you have to do one of those things. It is not good for you and it is not good for the baby to cut your time short. It was one more thing to add to our schedule and figure out how I was going to pump and travel and whatnot around when we could hold the boys, but it was more than worth it when we were finally able to hold them.

* * * * *

As amazing as it was to hold the boys for the first time, it was also surprisingly painful and uncomfortable for me. In order to hold the boys I had to take off my shirt and bra so that their cords would not get tangled in any of my clothing and allow for them to rest on my bare warm skin. The hospital provides (starchy, stiff and highly laundered) gowns that are worn backwards so your chest is exposed for the baby to lie on. I learned taking my bra off allowed the gown to rub against my nipples and cause both pain and milk to drip. Using LilyPadz® self-adhering nursing pads was the best solution I found to keep everything nice and secure so that holding the boys was painless. I put one pair in my hospital bag and had one pair at home so that I did not have to remember to pack them every day.

* * * * *

Pumping after holding your baby can stimulate you to provide more milk so it can be advantageous to time your pumping after you kangaroo care.

HOLDING THE BOYS WAS AMAZING AND ONLY got better as they slowly grew and were able to get rid of some of their gear. As they got bigger it was more and more enjoyable to hold them, to talk to them, and sing to them. It was fun to be able to hold them the first time they were able to wear clothes and the first time they were able to be swaddled. When the boys were lying against our chests, they were so small and their position had to be such that we could not see their faces while we held them. The nurses gave us hand mirrors to use to watch their faces when we held them. It was not only nice to be able to look at them, but it was also helpful if we had to adjust their vent or CPAP we could see how it looked.

* * * * *

Numerous studies have shown the effectiveness of skin-to-skin kangaroo care and of parents (specifically mother's) talking and singing to babies in the NICU. As wonderful as these things are for the parents to be able to do, they are medically advantageous for the babies as well. Babies who are held more and given kangaroo care do better and leave the NICU faster than babies that are not. Babies who hear their mother's voice during feeding have also been shown to leave the NICU sooner and eat more than babies that do not.

THE BOYS' VENT SETTINGS WENT UP AND down day after day for weeks. Some days it would seem as though they were doing more work on their own and then the next day they would have a bad gas and their settings would have to be turned back up. They both had minor infections here and there that required antibiotics, but luckily nothing became systemic and after a few doses they were back to acting like themselves. For a long time, it seemed as though they were only making baby steps in the right direction. It felt as though they would be in the hospital forever. I asked one of the nurses how long the longest stay she had seen was and she said the baby had had its first birthday party in the NICU. That was depressing but also a reality check. Even if our boys came home around their due date, that was still months away. Some days were very discouraging and it seemed like we were so far from where all the other babies were. It was hard not to compare our situation to others when I saw new babies being brought in looking so big and healthy compared to my guys. A few days later I saw those same babies leaving to go home. Thankfully we had our primary nurses to keep us informed of all the positive steps the boys took, even the tiny ones.

* * * * *

A lot of family and friends asked if we had made friends with other parents in the NICU. I know many people that remain friends with parents of babies who were in the NICU at the same time as their babies. We did not happen to have that experience. None of the other babies in our pod were there nearly as long as our boys were, so I saw a lot of parents come and go quickly. Others did not speak English when they visited and therefore we did not reach out to them because we assumed communication would be a problem. I did speak to one very young mom one night about her son, while we were waiting for the end of shift change to go visit, since I had overheard that he had been born at 24 weeks as well. She and I compared notes for a few minutes, and I enjoyed speaking with her and looked for her the next night. She did not visit during the day because she lived 3 hours away. Unfortunately, 2 days later her son was diagnosed with NEC also. It was very sudden and she was hysterical as the surgeon prepped for his procedure. My husband and I were about to leave from our weeknight visit, but I stayed with her as she waited the 3 hours for her mom to drive to the hospital to be with her. After an hour one of the other moms who she knew better arrived and took over sitting with her as she sobbed. It was heart wrenching to go home that night, but I promised I would visit with her in the morning and check on her son. The next day there was an empty space where her son's incubator was. For confidentiality reasons the nurses could not tell me what had happened, and I tried to think of reasons why he would not be there. There were no reasons other than he had not survived the surgery. For a long time I could not stop thinking about her and what she was going through and how similar our situations had been and yet how drastically different they became.

* * * * *

Primary nurses are nurses that your baby will be assigned every time that nurse is working. Babies who will be in the NICU a long time really benefit from primary nurses because those nurses get to know the baby and have an acute sense when something is off. We ended up with 5 primary nurses. A few we asked to sign up for one of the boys and a few signed up themselves after working with one of the boys a few days in a row. There were very few times during the day shift that one of our nurses was not one of our primaries. It was also reassuring to be able to call in the middle of the night and know that someone who really knew your baby was watching over them. We love our primary nurses. During the boys' NICU stay I talked to them a hundred times more than I talked to my family, to my friends, and most days, to my husband. When you are at the hospital for hours on end, day after day, they will become more than your nurse, more than a friend; they will become your family. Our primary called me to apologize because one of the boys pooped on his blanket and she could not rinse it all out. Our primary gave me her cell phone number because she was going to be on vacation when Chuck had his surgery and she wanted to be sure she heard as soon as possible that he came through it well. Our primary gave the boys gifts when they finally left the NICU. Our primaries called each other when they were not working to get an update on our boys. Our primaries insisted on being updated after we went home. They wanted photos and they shared them with doctors and other nurses. Our primary was our first baby sitter. There are no words to express how important our primaries are to us and how much we love them.

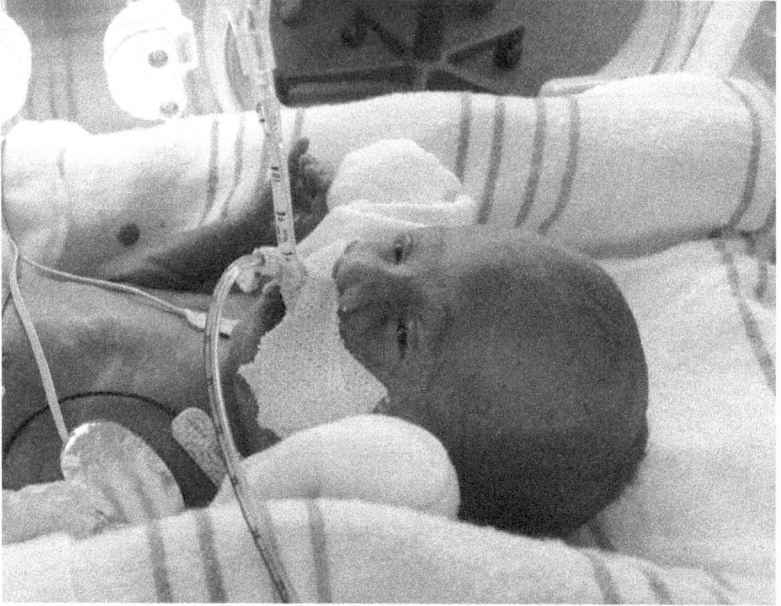

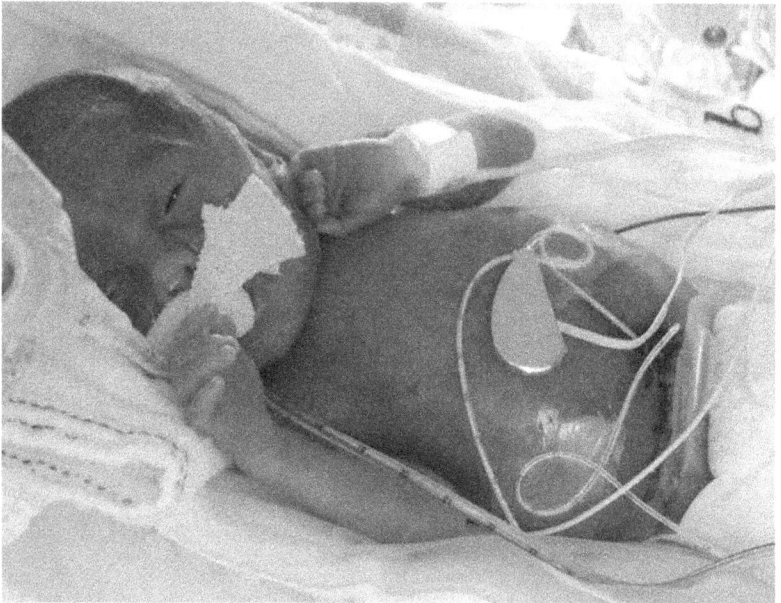

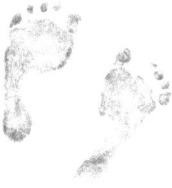

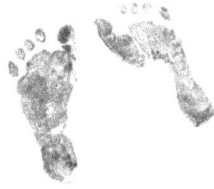

<u>Poop</u>

IT IS FAIRLY WELL KNOWN - POOP BECOMES very important in the NICU. After Chuck had his first surgery and got his ostomy, we played the waiting game for him to poop. Poop would come directly out of his intestine and into a bag that was secured to his abdomen with skin barrier powder and a wafer to protect the skin around his incision from the acidic and irritating juices that would be produced from it. Once he pooped, we would know that things were moving in the right direction from his stomach and out of his intestine. It would show that his intestines were healthy, were functioning well, and were moving things down and out properly. Once he pooped, he could resume breastmilk feedings through his OG tube.

Pedi Surg became concerned after a few days when he still had not pooped because that was longer than they had anticipated. They ordered a contrast study, which involved dye inserted through his stoma, with the goal of seeing it travel up his intestines and into his stomach on the X-ray. That would indicate the pathway through his intestines was all clear of any blockages or constrictions. Chuck went with the transport team to another floor to have the procedure done and did not tolerate it well. He needed extra oxygen during the procedure, and the transport team called a halt when they felt he became too stressed. Unfortunately, because they had to end early, they did not have enough time to get the dye all the way to his stomach. The x-ray did show that it went high enough that Pedi Surg was fairly confident that there was not a major problem. Because of that, he was able to start back on breastmilk the next day and we kept our fingers crossed that everything from the point where the dye stopped up to his stomach was actually clear and working as it should.

It was about this time, 2 months after they were born, that

the team was able to move Chuck to Henry's side of the room so that their incubators could be next to each other for the first time. They were both well over 2 pounds and were stable enough to finally share one nurse. That was a huge step in the right direction. It was great news that not only were they both doing well enough that one nurse could take care of both of them, but it also allowed me to talk to one nurse for an update instead of the nurses shuffling the cell phone between themselves on two sides of the pod every time I called. It was nice not to have to move my big backpack with my lunch, pumping equipment, dirty linen I was taking home to wash, and clean linen I was bringing in, along with a purse, all from one bedside to the next when I visited with the boys during the day.

* * * * *

Sometimes NICUs are divided between floors or wings of a hospital depending on what level of care a baby needs. Babies may be moved from one NICU to another or multiples may be split between NICUs. This can cause extra time and hassle when visiting.

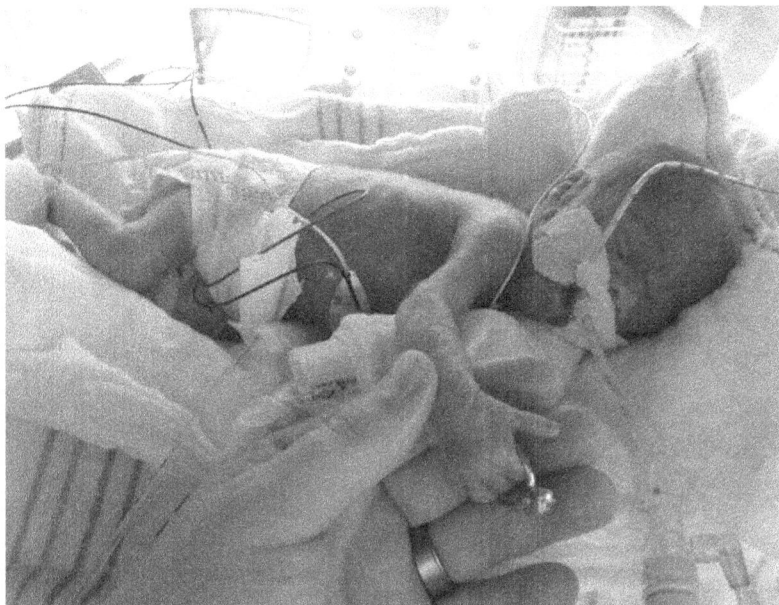

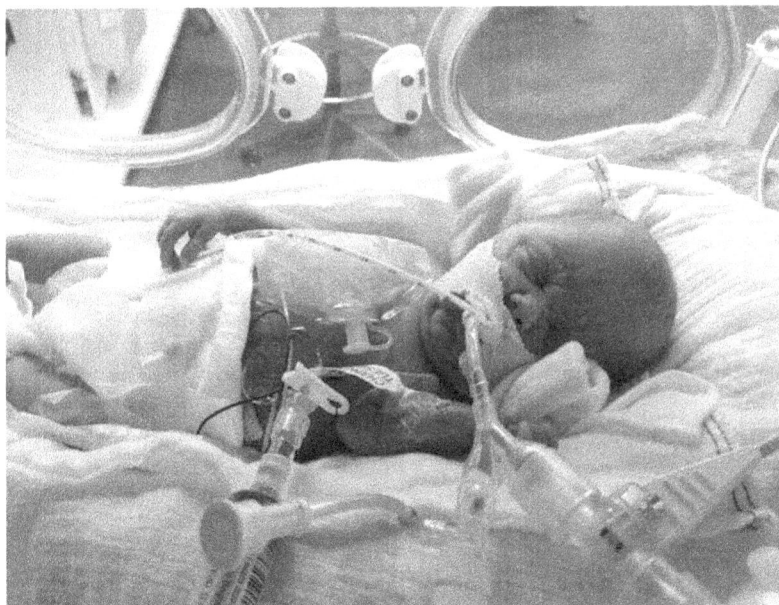

Tiny

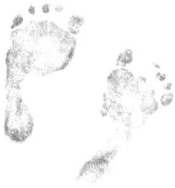

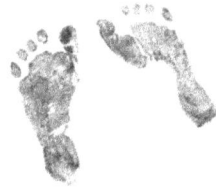

Studies

BOTH BOYS HAD BEEN ENROLLED IN A STUDY almost from the day they were both born. The study was not invasive to them; it involved the nurses putting a cotton ball in their diaper to collect urine and their vital signs being recorded. Of course it was voluntary, but we did not see a downside, which is why we enrolled them. When Chuck became more stable, we were able to enroll him in a Hydrocortisone study. Steroids are given to help decrease the time a baby needs to be on a vent. They are not without risks, but the risks from being on the vent for as long as the boys had been were beginning to outweigh the risks of the steroids themselves. Hydrocortisone is not the traditional steroid given for this purpose, so the study was trying to determine if it could offer the same benefits without as many risks as the more traditional steroid used. We were told that it would be fairly obvious if he was given the drug or the placebo because we should notice a marked improvement. If he got the drug, he would be able to be weaned off the vent fairly quickly. He would begin to have great gases, one after another, and his settings could be turned down until he no longer needed a vent. However, after a few days his settings did not change much and we assumed he had been given the placebo. That was disappointing. Henry was also enrolled in two additional studies. Surfactant is a drug given for lung development and was given to the boys as soon as they were born. Henry's study questioned whether or not additional surfactant, given later on, could help babies get off the vent. He was also given nitric oxide during a study determining if it was helpful to babies on vents. Although we did not notice much of a change during his time in the study, hopefully the results will help neonatologists in the future.

* * * * *

Studies are always optional. We felt there little to no risk in the studies in which the boys were enrolled and hoped that the trial drugs would have a positive effect. Our neonatologists always assured us that if they felt something was causing a baby any harm, or if a different medication or procedure was needed, they would stop the study drug and give the medication or perform the procedure. The health of the baby always trumps the study if there is a conflict. Some medications cannot be given while a baby is enrolled in a study, but if the baby needs that medication they are simply unenrolled in the study. We hope that what was learned from our boys will help make decisions easier for future NICU babies. Once the boys were discharged, we simply had to answer some questions over the phone every few months and bring the boys in for a quick physical a few times before they turned two.

* * * * *

While your baby is in the NICU, you may be approached by a physician or nurse coordinating a study for which your baby qualifies. It can be helpful to speak to your baby's primary nurse or the neonatologist fellow or attending about what they feel the benefit would be to your baby. The person coordinating the study will let you know how long you have to make a decision and can answer any questions you have. They should also let you know the requirements for follow up and what you might receive as compensation. After each study ended, we received a gift card to Walmart for compensation.

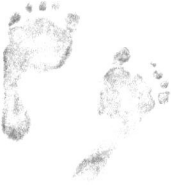

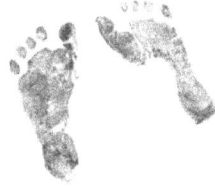

Growing Boys

BECAUSE THE BOYS HAD GROWN SO MUCH (over a pound in weight is a lot to put on!), they were able to get new vent tubes. These were larger in diameter and they filled more of their airways. The boys had been having problems with their vents "leaking," meaning a certain amount of air was getting forced into their lungs but some of it would seep back up around their tube and out of their mouth. Therefore, they were not actually getting the full dose of oxygen the machine was trying to give them. Larger tubes filled up more of this space and decreased the amount that could leak out. As soon as they got new tubes, their vents were turned down to reflect how much oxygen they required and not how much they needed plus whatever leaked out around their tubes. It can be very tricky to reintubate such a tiny baby to place a new larger tube. Because one of our primary nurses had the boys that day, she called me after the tubes were placed and everything had gone well instead of beforehand so I could avoid sweating and holding my breath until I heard that things had gone well. Luckily everything went smoothly.

Because Henry was doing so well, up to full feeds of breastmilk (fortified for extra calories) through his OG tube and no longer needing TPN as additional nutrition, he was able to have his PICC line removed. It was a great feeling that he was able to have one more line removed. It was also difficult to have one baby doing so well and another struggling. Chuck was having a hard time tolerating the TPN and breastmilk. Breastmilk can cause babies with an ostomy to not digest all they need from the milk and produce too much watery stool (dumping). It was very difficult to celebrate going up in quantity on his breastmilk and down on the TPN only to hear he was having a lousy day dumping and to go back to square one. He had to be a certain weight, and otherwise stable, to have his reversal surgery. In theory, once he had the reversal to reconnect his intestine and reinsert it into his abdomen, his entire length of his intestines would be used to properly absorb nutrition from breastmilk and he would gain weight normally without dumping. However, he had to gain weight before the surgery to be big enough and not have the entire length of his bowel to absorb nutrition and gain weight with.

Gaining weight on TPN can be a very long process and is not without its own risks. Babies (or people) are not meant to live on TPN. Chuck got all the way to full breastmilk feeds with no TPN, only to get an infection and retain a lot of fluid. He looked very puffy for a long time. At one point his little face was so puffy his eyes could not open. He was put on diuretics to try to get rid of some of that extra fluid. He was finally in a good place and not dumping as much, and even had his PICC line out. Then his blood pH started measuring too acidic and his liver looked large, indicating it was working too hard, there was an infection, or the change to breastmilk had been too quick for him to adjust. All of this meant he needed to go back onto the TPN, which meant he had to have a PICC line put back in. It was very discouraging. The nurses even talked to me about what it would mean if we could not get him to gain enough weight and he was stable enough to go home but with the ostomy. Although I felt confident I could learn how to care for a stoma if I had to, I was very much hoping he would be able to have the reversal surgery before he came home from the hospital.

Chuck went through weeks of increasing the breastmilk only to start dumping and having to increase TPN and decrease breastmilk again and again for multiple attendings. It was the goal of each attending to get him off TPN and back to breastmilk. However, each time we tried he would start dumping and fail to gain weight. He was simply not making enough progress quickly enough towards reaching to the 2000 grams (4.4 pounds) weight he needed to be for his reversal surgery. On the first day of a new attending, one of his nurses asked specifically that I be there for rounds to explain his pattern to the new attending and ask what she thought about keeping him on the 50/50 TPN/breastmilk combo until he finally reached the goal weight and could have the surgery. She agreed to put the new plan in place to leave him where he was with his nutrition until he reached the weight he needed to be for his reversal surgery rather than again trying to reach full feeds on breastmilk. His nurses and I were relieved; we thought we had a good plan and he could reach the goal.

* * * * *

Everyone on your baby's team certainly has the baby's best interest in mind, but you are your baby's advocate. It is your job (along with your baby's primary nurses as your allies) to voice your opinion. That does not mean you know more than your baby's neonatologist, but it means you have a valid position to be heard. More than once everyone was glad to have my input and I was glad I had been there to offer it. Make sure you are heard so that the team around your baby can do the best things possible to get your baby home.

WE WERE EXTREMELY LUCKY TO HAVE ONE of the best ophthalmologists in the country scanning the boys for ROP. She checked the boys' eyes between 31 and 32 weeks of what should have been their gestation but was actually week 5 of their life after birth. After seeing Henry a few times over a few weeks, she was able to clear him of ROP and predict he would have no lasting problems because of the oxygen he was on due to his prematurity. Chuck, however, was diagnosed with Stage 2 (of 5) ROP. His ophthalmologist thought this was probably due to the unavoidably high concentration of oxygen he had required during his first surgery. Later stages of ROP require an injection to the eye or surgery to prevent blood vessels from forming incorrectly and possibly leading to blindness. She said 95% of the time this does the trick, but sometimes a second shot is required, which she said always give the result she looks for. Chuck was seen every week and then every 2 weeks until his ophthalmologist was finally convinced he was not going to progress to Stage 3. It was a relief that we could continue to follow him but were not concerned with long term vision issues due to the ROP.

Tiny

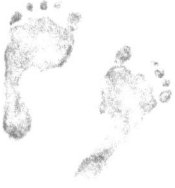

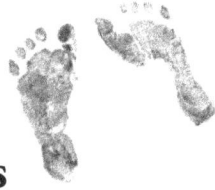

Weekend Visits

DRIVING TO AND FROM THE HOSPITAL EVERY day by myself for my morning visit usually involved trying to avoid traffic while also arriving in time for rounds. Some attendings held rounds later in the morning so I could leave the house after morning traffic and be there in time to listen. However, some began earlier and I had to leave before traffic. This meant sometimes I left the house at 5 am, usually waking up, pumping and showering before I left. On the weekends my husband and I visited together so we got to share the ride down and back and rounds were later in the day. Because Children's Memorial Hermann is located in a great part of Houston, we were relatively new to the area and had not explored very much, and it was almost an hour drive each way, we used the weekend trips to go out to lunch either before or after our visit. It helped to extend the time to not feel like we were doing as much driving as we actually were and to give us something nice to do away from the hospital.

By the time the boys were big enough and doing well enough to be held, we could each hold a baby and do kangaroo care at the same time. Because of how the cords and leads and everything was situated on one side or the other of the incubator and plugged into or near the wall and such, we did not always sit on the same side of the incubators. That meant sometimes we could not even really see each other while we held one of the boys, but by that time we were spending every Saturday and Sunday driving down and back together and every weekday night driving down and back together so it was not the end of the world to be separated by an incubator while we held a baby for a few hours. Some of the nurses tried to make the wires work for us to sit together, and it was nice that a few months into our NICU journey we were able to take our first family photo with all four of us.

* * * * *

It is okay to incorporate other things into visits to the hospital. For a long time I felt like we had to hurry up and get to the NICU, stay as long as possible, and then go home and do nothing else enjoyable or else we were bad parents. It made the trips more pleasant and relaxing when we started adding in lunch or dinner somewhere as a treat for us on weekend days.

WE WERE REALLY GETTING TO KNOW OUR nurses on the weekends as well as during the week. I spent all my time with them during the week, but since their schedules vary and there are not 'weekday nurses' or 'weekend nurses' we saw them on weekends as well. During one of our weekend visits in the middle of the summer while two of our primaries were working, I started getting very cold. I never got to hold the boys as much as my husband on weekends because I had to pump as soon as we got to the hospital and before we left while he was able to just visit. He got to start holding while I was pumping and finish while I was pumping. One particular day when I was finishing pumping and we were almost ready to leave, I started to shiver in my t-shirt. I thought it was because I had not remembered to bring a sweatshirt. When I got back to the boys' pod, I wrapped up in one of the quilts we had brought to cover the incubators with. Once something touches the floor in the NICU it needs to be laundered, so even though something may be clean if it hits the floor it has to be taken home and washed. I wrapped up in this quilt that had touched the floor and was on its way home with us. I started feeling pretty crappy on the drive home as well. I had not been sick in years and it took a while to finally realize I might have a temperature. I mentioned this to my husband and when we got home I took my temperature and it was 103.6. Well that's not good, I thought.

Since it was a Saturday I could not make a same day appointment with my OB/GYN, but being only 7 weeks postpartum I was worried I could have some sort of uterine infection. Since those infections can get serious quite quickly, we decided it could not wait until Monday. We drove to a stand-alone Urgent Care center down the street. When I told them I was 7 weeks postpartum and had a fever, they let me know they would not treat me but that the private emergency room next door could. We went out one door and in the other and were informed that my insurance would not cover a visit there the same way it would at a traditional hospital emergency room. Since we knew what our copay was at an actual hospital emergency room, and were worried the stand-alone emergency room would be at least that much or more, we decided to go to the emergency room at the hospital. I was seen quite quickly and since my temperature was now 104.2, the emergency room doctor was concerned. I had blood drawn and an exam and everything seemed to be normal. Luckily, as fate would have it, my nurse was a mom of twins herself and had breastfed her babies. When she heard I was pumping and had a fever, she immediately asked to look at my breasts. She felt a big lump in one and asked if it was painful. As soon as she pointed it out I realized that it had been uncomfortable, but I had been trying to massage it when I pumped thinking it was something normal. Hearing that she immediately told the doctor she was quite confident that it was the problem. He agreed with her that I had a bad case of mastitis; a common infection breastfeeding moms can get that can be quickly treated with a strong antibiotic. He prescribed one I could take while continuing to pump.

I was in and out of the emergency room in under an hour. We were very relieved I did not have something more serious. Since I do not get sick often, my body reacts very quickly to antibiotics and I was looking forward to feeling better as soon as we got the prescription filled on our way home. Once in the car I realized I had not asked whether or not the milk I had already pumped at the hospital was okay to give the boys. We called the NICU on the way home and one of our two primary nurses who we had left a few hours before answered. I let her know I was leaving the emergency room with an antibiotic for mastitis and wondered if the milk I had already pumped was safe. I could hear her conversation with our other primary and how she could not believe we ended up in the emergency room after just seeing us. We all had a good laugh at my misfortune and luckily she told me the milk was fine.

The NICU (thankfully, for the babies' sake) did not allow anyone that was ill or had a fever to visit. That meant that when I woke up the next day, even though I felt better and knew there was no way I could make my or anyone else's babies ill I could not go in and see the boys because I still had a fever. I am a rule follower, through and through. But I also could not bear to let my husband drive down by himself and visit the boys without me while I stayed at home and did "nothing" at home. I went to the Ronald McDonald House™ lounge and sat on the couch while my husband went in to visit and hold one of the boys. I went to the pumping room to pump and peaked at the boys through the window on my way back to the lounge. One of our primary nurses came in to see me. Technically the nurses are not supposed to be in the Ronald McDonald House™ area. The Ronald McDonald House™ tries to maintain a non-medical safe haven for parents and families. However, no one else was around so she came to give me an update on the boys since I could not touch them with my own two hands that day. That meant a lot.

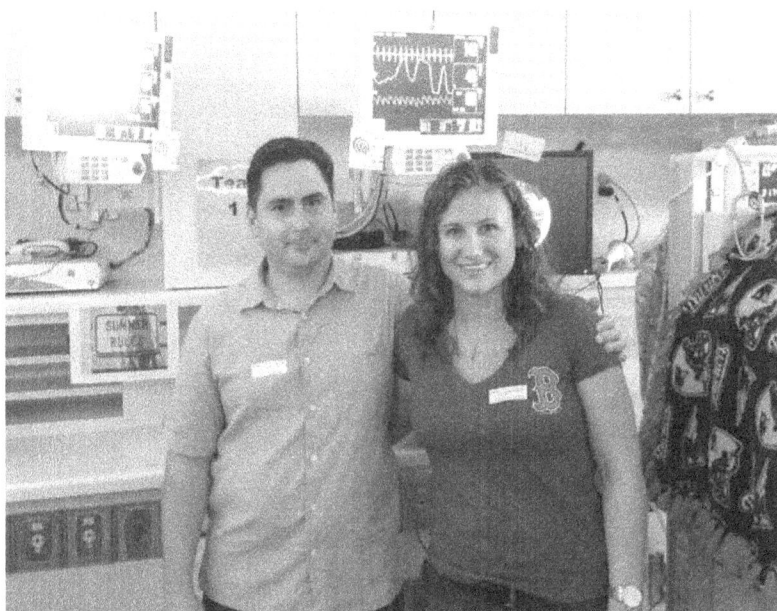

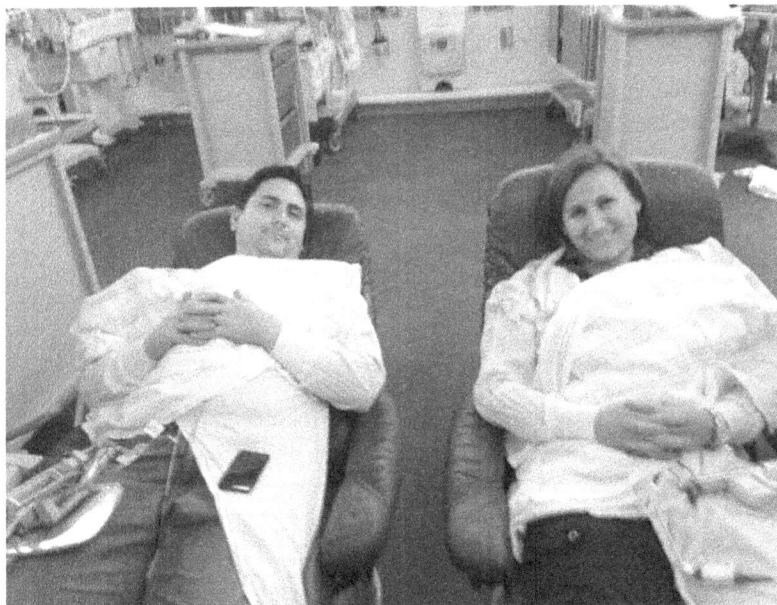

Tiny

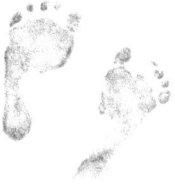

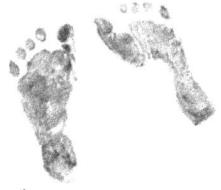

Finally Getting Off the Vents

THE BOYS WERE MAKING SOME PROGRESS with their vent settings in a positive direction, but not as much as they needed to in order to reassure the doctors that they would be able to breathe on their own within a few weeks. The steroid given to help babies breathe on their own has risks, but so does staying on the vent for extremely prolonged periods of time. The boys were now going on day 57 on vents. Conversations with their nurses had changed from hoping the boys would not need the steroid and wanting to give them more time to show progress and come off the vents on their own to the nurses deciding they were going to push for the steroid in rounds and let the doctor know that the boys' progress recently was too little and too late. This was one instance of initially dreading a medication and ending up looking forward to it. The boys were given caffeine to prepare them for the inevitability of receiving the steroid. Caffeine gave them just enough of a kick to remind them to breathe when they no longer had the vent to rely on. It also allowed me to have my first caffeinated beverage since I became pregnant. I was adamant about only putting the best things into my body to grow the boys and produce milk for them, but when they were getting caffeine shots I decided I could have a little too.

* * * * *

It is hard to manage expectations when things are constantly changing with your baby. I think it helped that we were never 100% opposed to anything the doctors or nurses talked about and it helped that when we were informed of things possibly on the horizon we were always given the pros and the cons. There are side effects to everything. If you start with the mindset that you are totally against a medication or surgery, it may be very difficult if all of a sudden the doctors are telling you that it is the only thing that will help your baby. Although steroids come with their own risks, we had known they were a possibility so we were prepared that the boys may need them.

* * * * *

It may or may not be helpful for friends and family to research on their own and present questions about drugs or procedures to parents. Every hospital is different, so telling someone with a very sick child that you have heard of this new thing at another hospital or that another baby benefited from may not be helpful if parents ask about it and are told it would not be appropriate for their baby or is not something that is done in their hospital. Many people commented on how co-bedding twins was such a help to someone they know, only to be disappointed when I told them our boys would never be in the same incubator. Not only did our hospital subscribe to the American Association of Pediatrics guideline that the possible negative consequences of co-sleeping twins outweigh the benefits and so as a policy it does not co-bed siblings, but our guys had so many wires and leads and tubes that it would have been a nightmare to keep everything straight if the boys had been together in the same incubator. Also, at least initially, the boys were so fragile that it was difficult enough for a nurse to get her or his hands in and out without jostling them or their vent tube. To add another baby to the same incubator would not have made sense. It still felt as though we were disappointing people when they asked about them sleeping together and we told them it was not going to happen.

FINALLY THE BOYS WERE GIVEN THEIR FIRST dose of the steroid. The expectation and the hope was that their nurses would begin getting great gases and be able to, fairly consistently and quickly, wean their settings down until they no longer needed the vent and could be extubated. The steroid was given in decreasing concentrations over the course of 8 days. The goal was extubation on or before day 5, for there still to be a few days of medication that would assist the boys when they were breathing on their own. When I called the night nurse at 2 am, the boys had been on the steroid about 12 hours and I was very excited to hear that they had made some prog-ress. We were looking forward to hearing how they had done for the rest of the night when we visited the next day.

When we arrived for our weekend afternoon visit, the recep-tionist called down to see if we could go back to our pod and was told that a new baby was just getting settled so we would need to wait a few minutes before going back to visit. We hung out in the waiting room for about 10 minutes before being told we could go on back. When we walked in, two of the boys' primary nurses, their nurse practitioner and their respiratory therapist were standing in the cen-ter of the room. I put down my backpack full of pumping supplies and proceeded to open it and start to put away clean linen before I took a peak at the boys. As I was putting things away, my husband let out a gasp. I went over to one of the incubators and was shocked to see there was no vent tube coming out of Chuck's mouth. There was no vent tube coming out of Henry's mouth either. Instead of taking 3-5 days to be extubated, both boys took less than 24 hours. Our nurses had made up an excuse to keep us out of the pod to finish extubating and surprise us with vent-less boys. It was pretty hard to believe. Everyone had big smiles and told us how well the boys had done. It was also exciting because it was the first time we could see all of Henry and Chuck's mouths and some of their cheeks.

* * * * *

Lots of babies need help breathing in some form or another at various points during their NICU stay. It is important to remember, however, that if they have made progress to a less invasive breathing machine they may at some point require more help and go back. We had some yo-yo time with Chuck going back and forth between the oscillating vent and the regular vent. Babies sometimes come off a vent and need to go back on when they become too tired breathing on their own. It can be very disappointing. It is important to remember that the baby needs all its energy to grow and sometimes breathing on its own can be so tiring that it prevents the baby from good sleep and growth.

BEING OFF A VENTILATOR CAN MEAN A LOT of different things for a baby. For our boys, it did not mean that they could breathe completely on their own. They were still very far from that. But they could do enough of the work that they could be on a CPAP instead of the vent. Because the CPAP does not involve a tube down their throat, we now had the opportunity to hear the boys cry for the first time. It would seem strange for a lot of people to be waiting for their two month old baby to cry for the first time. The boys' CPAP consisted of a felt hat that held a soft rubber pronged tube to each nostril to keep pressurized air blowing down their throat. The positive pressure was just enough help to remind them to breathe and the CPAP could also give additional oxygen if necessary.

The CPAP was taken off for a few minutes every few hours for the nurse to check it, give the boys' noses a little massage, and reposition their hats. The first time I saw the nurse take the CPAP off one of the boys I was terrified that he would stop breathing. I kept my eyes on the monitor the whole time to make sure he was still taking breaths and his oxygen saturation was above where it needed to be. I was sure the oxygen concentration would plummet and he would need to be bagged. I was shocked at how well he actually did breathing on his own. It had not occurred to me he could actually breathe on his own for a period of time. I also realized that because I had my eyes on the monitor I had missed seeing Chuck's entire face, unencumbered, for the very first time. The next time the CPAP was removed I made sure to take a photo of each of our boys' entire face to show friends and family. It was actually very strange to see their whole faces for the first time after only seeing bits and pieces of them for months. The first time I ever saw Henry's whole face was in a photo my husband texted me while I was in the pumping room.

Getting off the vents was such a big step in the right direction that I asked a nurse when she guessed the boys would be coming home. Typically, right around the baby's due date is a good ballpark date for babies to leave the NICU. When the boys got off their vents, their due date was still almost 8 weeks away. In our case, however, since Chuck was still having trouble gaining weight, she guessed he would need an additional month over Henry before he came home.

This was the first time it occurred to my husband that the boys would not necessarily come home at the same time. I had known other moms who had twins in the NICU and so I had known that it was a distinct possibility. However, it was disappointing to us both to think that it was now very probable that we would take one baby home and leave one at the hospital.

* * * * *

Many times multiples are ready to leave the NICU at different times, which allows for a slower transition into actually caring for multiples alone at home without doctors and nurses. It can be heart wrenching to leave one baby "alone" at the hospital. I heard many times "Oh, this is actually a good thing; now you can see what it's like to take care of one baby before the other one comes home!" That was hard to hear. No, this was not a good thing. Having a baby so sick they still needed to be in the NICU was not a good thing. Turning a very bad situation into a positive is not always what parents want to hear. It would have been much more helpful to have heard "Now you'll have one baby at home and one in the NICU...how can we help?" It is pretty obvious it is easier to take care of only one baby at home and not two; I did not need to be told that. Add the stress of a second baby in the NICU to taking care of one baby at home and it was too hard to hear that it was "a good thing."

* * * * *

Babies coming home at different times can drastically affect how parents visit the NICU. All NICUs have certain rules on visiting with siblings. At ours, the minimum age for siblings to visit was too old for us to bring Henry to visit after he came home. Our NICU also had a "no repeat customers" policy, as one nurse told me. By definition a hospital is a place for sick people, and the last place you want to bring an infant who was recently discharged from the NICU is to a place full of sick people. Therefore, as much as they want to see discharged siblings doing well, they do not want to see them back in the NICU visiting. This made complete sense. However, having to be home to care for one baby meant that I could no longer visit during the day and my husband and I could no longer visit at night together. We made the tentative plan that we would take turns every night if one baby came home before the other. Either my husband would leave from work and visit the NICU before coming home or he would come home so that I could leave the house and visit. That way we could make sure the baby in the hospital never went a day without a long visit from one of us.

* * * * *

Having one baby at home and one in the NICU can be extremely rough emotionally for a lot of reasons. It was actually hard to revel in the joy of having one baby home because I felt guilty about being so happy at home with another baby in the NICU. I felt awful that all day would go by without a parent there at the hospital to be with Chuck. It helped that by the time we were in this situation we had gotten to know our primary nurses so well that we knew that if we could not be there they were the next best thing.

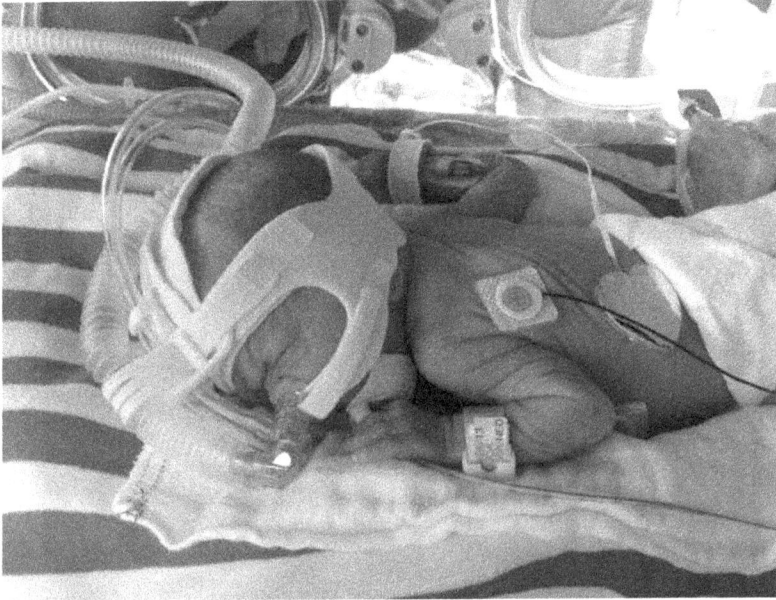

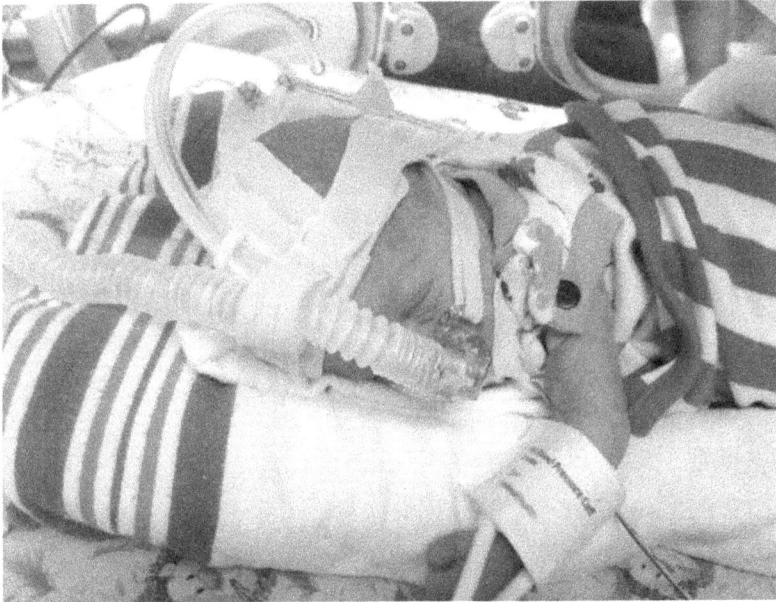

Tiny

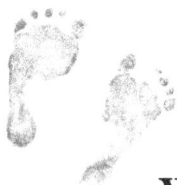

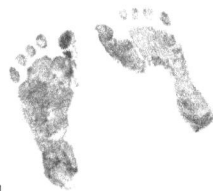

When One Does Well and One Does Not

IT IS VERY HARD TO HAVE TWO SICK BABIES in the NICU. It is harder to have one sick baby and one sicker baby in the NICU. Although both boys were making great progress on the CPAP and requiring less and less pressure to keep them breathing on their own, Chuck was still having a lot of trouble gaining weight and lots of days where he was dumping out of his ostomy. One of our attendings suggested that I change my pumping strategy to help him more. I was ready to do anything I could, and I made the changes he suggested immediately. Breastmilk is more calorically dense and contains more fat during the second half of a baby's nursing time or pumping time than the first half. The second 12 minutes of what I pumped contained more fat and calories than the first 12 minutes. Ideally, Chuck needed as much fat and as many calories as we could give him and the fat and calories in breastmilk were the best kind he could receive (he was also getting corn oil and other additives). Every time I pumped I took the second 12 minutes and labeled and packaged that milk for Chuck and took the first 12 minutes and labeled it to take home. I did not want Henry to have fewer calories and fat than regular breastmilk so I did not want it given to him, but I was also chastised (read-nicely yelled at) by the NICU nurses when they learned I had thrown away the first half. Although it was not ideal for Henry while he was in the hospital, that first half (we called it "skim") could be used later when the boys were much bigger and healthier when even breastmilk with slightly less fat and calories than regular breastmilk would be better for them than anything else. This became my new routine for pumping. It took more time and effort, but we hoped it would make a positive impact on Chuck's weight gain.

Henry, in the meantime, weighed so much (1500 grams or a whopping 3 pounds 5 ounces) and was doing so well holding his own temperature without warm air blowing into the incubator that he was allowed to wear clothes for the first time and try an open crib. An open crib does not provide the warm air that the boys had initially received in the incubator, and additionally it does not offer protection from the drafts of the fairly chilly NICU. It turned out Henry did not love the crib and he was back in an incubator very quickly because he was not able to keep his temperature high enough. He had also been doing so well on the CPAP, even deciding he did not need it and pushing it out of his nose without setting off any alarms when he lay on his tummy. He, therefore, was given a nasal cannula instead of the CPAP. The cannula gave him additional oxygen but no additional pressure to keep his airway open, so his lungs were now doing all the work. That, combined with having to work to maintain his temperature in the open crib, had tired him out and his vitals showed it. It was much more important to keep him breathing on his own and gaining weight than wasting energy to keep warm. By the next day all the hard work had taken a toll and he was back on the CPAP in the incubator. But it was a good first try, and all our nurses said it was not the end of the world and we would let him get a little bigger over the next week and try again.

* * * * *

Breathing and maintaining temperature is hard work for little babies. Many times there will be a period of time going back and forth between CPAP and cannula or crib and incubator. For the most part, these are minor things that micro preemies and preemies are faced with mastering. Most of the time it is a matter of when, and not if, babies master these skills, so do not get too discouraged when there are setbacks.

BRADYCARDIA EVENTS (BRADYS) ARE ANOTHER constant in the NICU for very small babies. Bradys happen when the baby's heart rate drops below 80 beats per minute. Breathing apnea is another event that goes along with bradys and breathing issues. Apnea is when the baby stops breathing for longer than 20 seconds. This usually causes a brady and sets off their alarms. During rounds the doctors and nurses would talk about the boys' "As and Bs" and discuss how many events of Apnea and Bradycardia they had in the last 24 hours and how they were handled. Sometimes it just took a few seconds and the baby would take a big breath and the heartbeat would go back to normal on its own. Sometimes they needed a little rub on their foot or back to wake them a bit and remind them to breathe and then their heartbeat would return to normal. Other times they would need a few additional breaths given by the push of a button on the vent or they would need to be bagged. When a baby gets bagged it looks awful, like something you see on T.V when an oxygen mask is put over someone's face or it is attached to a vent tube and breaths are pushed into the bag.

The first time Henry needed to be bagged we were walking in for a weekend visit and saw some commotion at his incubator and two nurses standing over him. One was holding the bag to the end of his vent tube that came out of his mouth and giving him additional breaths. Since we had never seen this before and it looked serious, we asked what was wrong and I will never forget his nurse saying, in a voice so calm, "Oh, he just needed some extra breaths." We asked if she had tried using the vent to give them, as we had seen before. She said, "He didn't seem to like that...he's coming back now...here he is," as his heartbeat and color returned to normal. When a baby needs to be bagged, it is fairly serious and they usually have a pale face and a bit of a blue tinge to their lips because they are not getting enough oxygen. His nurse was so calm and acting as though it were nothing because she did it so often, which was reassuring to us. Luckily our guys did not need to be bagged too often, but in the beginning they needed extra breaths or their backs rubbed to get their breathing and heart rates back to normal quite a bit. It is not safe for a baby to still have As and Bs at home without monitors or support; therefore, the goal is to have outgrown them before babies are discharged. Of course the monitors let the nurses know when an apnea or brady event is happening and they were buzzing and dinging quite often because of our two guys.

At first it is very scary when alarms and buzzers go off, but as you get to know the monitors and your babies they become less scary.

The nurses can also silence the monitor while they are dealing with the problem so it does not continue to ding while they are handling the situation. Toward the end of our stay the boys were able to get their heart rates back on their own when they had their few last bradys and it was not very worrisome. Once I even silenced a monitor so that we did not have to continue to listen to it after one of the boys' heart rates came back up to normal because the nurse was on the other side of the room. As soon as I had pushed the button, I realized that it probably was not something I should be doing and turned around to tell the nurse what I had done. She just laughed. By this point we knew each other well.

* * * * *

There will come a point when the monitors and their noises are not so scary and do not send you into a panic every time they go off. Remember that any visitors who come with you to the NICU may not be familiar with the monitors and their sounds. Visitors can be much more on edge than parents and tend to panic at every sound. It is not great to bring added stress to the visit, and it can be helpful to remind friends or family that nurses deal with all emergencies quickly and efficiently and there is no need to bring more alarm to the situation.

* * * * *

When visiting, it can be hard not to be jumpy and panic at every alarm. It is important to be calm, especially when holding a baby. It can be helpful to remind yourself that if there really is a problem the nurse will come take care of it and let you know what you need to do, if anything. Unless the nurse needs your help, you can simply enjoy holding the baby.

BOTH BOYS WENT BACK AND FORTH FROM cannula, which only supplies additional oxygen just under their nose, to CPAP and back again as they got used to breathing more on their own. Going back and forth affected their weights a bit. The CPAP apparatus weighs more than the cannula does and they were weighed with it attached. Therefore, going from the vent to the CPAP and going from the CPAP to the cannula affected the nightly weigh in. It did not affect Henry as much because as long as he showed steady growth every few days we were not concerned with no gain or a small loss one particular night. His overall trend had always been continual weight gain. With Chuck it was more of a big deal. He was still trying to get to the 2000 grams for his reversal surgery and every little gram counted. When he would go from CPAP to cannula, it would show no gain or a loss. Even if we knew the underlying reason had to do with equipment weight it was still disappointing. We also noticed some nights when we were there he would gain a startlingly large amount. One of his nurses and I realized the scale he was being weighed on was making a difference so we tried to make sure he was weighed on the same one every night. Some incubators have built-in scales but some do not. Over the course of their stay, the boys had a few different incubators and the last they were in did not have built-in scales. It helped to try to keep track of "his" scale for his weigh-ins to be as accurate as possible as he tried to reach his goal weight.

During this time of going from CPAP to cannula and back again, I remembered that the hospital had different kinds of CPAP masks. The very first time the boys had gone to CPAP from their vents their primary nurse had made sure to get the mask that had two prongs that fit fairly tightly into their nostrils. That type of mask ensured all the pressurized air was getting up their nose and into their lungs and not slipping out underneath the mask. She knew it would give them the best chance of success on the CPAP without having to go back to the vent. After a few weeks, however, Chuck's nostrils were getting irritated from the back and forth from the cannula to CPAP and it was making him pretty unhappy. The unhappier he was, the worse his vitals were. He would get stuffy and bleed when his nose was cleaned. Then it would scab over but bleed again the next time it was irrigated and suctioned. I asked about the second type of mask that could be used with the CPAP and his nurse immediately got one. The new mask looked a lot more like a traditional oxygen mask you would put over your mouth and nose but shaped just for the nose. When she switched Chuck to this, he stopped fussing about the prongs being in his nostrils and his nose healed up quickly. With him being more comfortable, he could relax and put all his energy into gaining weight.

* * * * *

Major changes are usually made during the week and not on weekends. Sometimes on a weekend your baby's regular attending neonatologist is not working. Other attendings are less likely to make changes with babies they do not know as well. Sometimes this can be frustrating if there is a change you feel that needs to be made. We found that a more cautious approach with major changes made by those doctors and nurses who knew our boys best usually worked in our favor.

* * * * *

Do not be afraid to suggest something different that your baby seemed to prefer. You know your baby best and your suggestions should be taken seriously. I was glad I did not sit back and watch Chuck become frustrated and uncomfortable with the pronged CPAP mask. He was certainly glad I remembered the alternative and asked about it. You may feel that if there were something that could help the doctors or nurses would have already thought of it, but nurses and neonatologists take care of so many babies that every once in a while your suggestion could be one they wish they had thought of.

* * * * *

If you notice something you think is off, such as a scale or something else that may be inconsequential to another baby but important to yours, make sure you speak up. It took a couple nights of me really making a stink to different night nurses, but eventually everyone realized Chuck needed to be weighed on the same scale every night. Afterwards, everyone tried to be as consistent as possible.

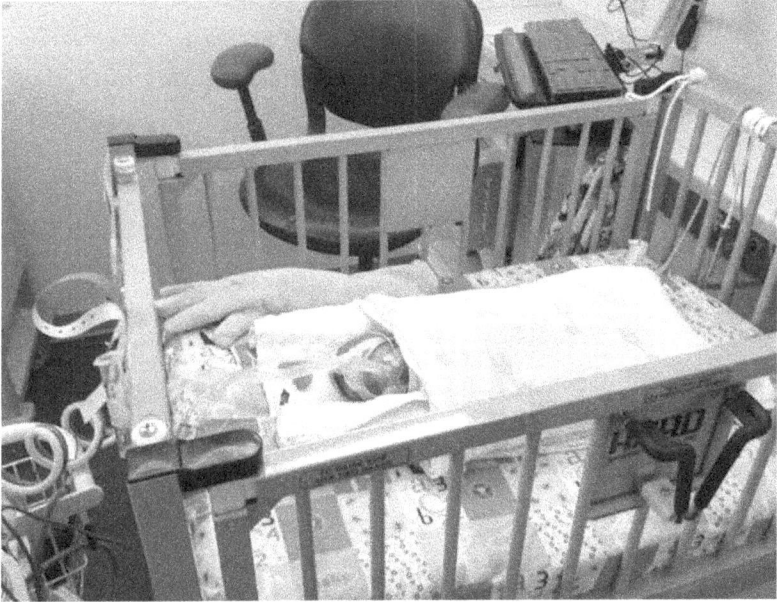

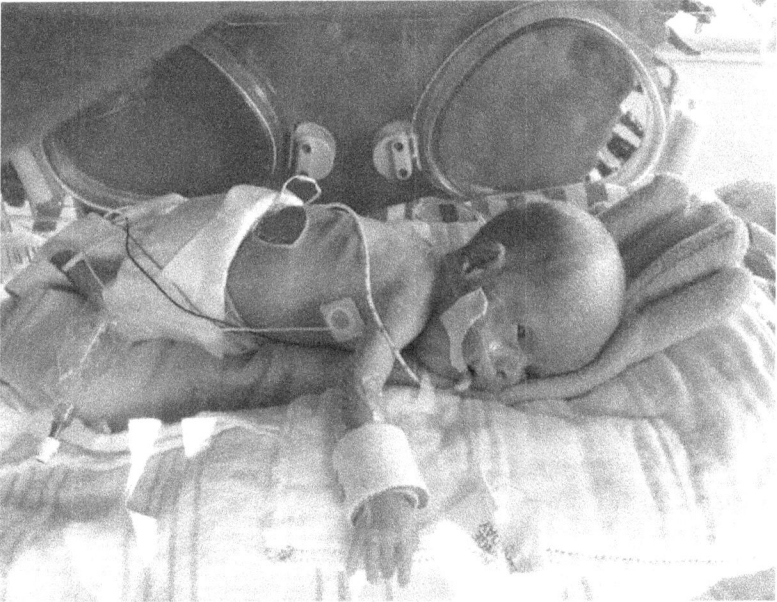

Tiny

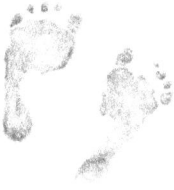

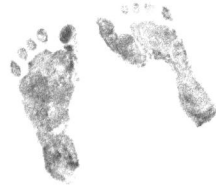

<u>Feeding</u>

FINALLY THE BOYS WERE DOING WELL ON the cannula and able to try to drink from a bottle for the first time. Since I wanted to breastfeed I tried that too, but mostly the boys received bottles so their nurses could track exactly how much they ate. The boys had been on a feeding schedule, receiving breastmilk through their OG tube every 3 hours. They stuck to that schedule with bottle feeding, even when it meant waking them up. If they fell asleep or got too tired and could not finish a bottle or their heart rate went up and they became exhausted and could not finish, the boys were given the remainder through their OG tube. Babies have to be consistently gaining weight and able to finish a certain number of bottles and a certain amount of milk every day for a number of days in a row before they can go home. We started off slow with one bottle a day and increased both the number of bottles a day and the amount in each bottle slowly as they tolerated it. Henry went first since he was more stable and heavier. It was a process since Henry was a baby who technically should still be in the womb and here we were expecting him to learn to suck, swallow and breathe at the same time. Babies who spend a lot of time on ventilators can have more trouble learning to do all those things at the same time than others.

* * * * *

Try different kinds of bottles if the NICU allows for it. Henry had some trouble at first, and a feeding specialist came by to evaluate him and gave us a different position to try as well as suggesting Dr. Brown's® bottles. We went out that night to buy the bottles to try them the next day and they, along with the new position, made a big difference. The specialist advised buying a few of whatever kind of bottle you are trying until you decide that the baby likes it.

* * * * *

The nurses have enough to do without washing your special bottles. Typically they use premixed formula or thawed breastmilk in disposable bottles/nipples. If you are using different bottles, try to take some of the burden off them. I made sure we had at least 24 hours' worth of bottles at the hospital so that my husband or I could clean what was dirty during our visit and the nurses would never have to clean any. I also brought in a bottle brush and a small bottle of dish detergent to keep right by their bedside to clean them with. I had one 2 gallon size zip top bag on which I wrote "dirty" for the nurses to toss the bottles in when they were finished with the feeds for which we were not at the hospital so I could clean the bottles during my visit. One of the staff made the comment at one point that they have a "love/hate relationship" with Dr. Brown's® bottles, and after the cleaning requirements and all that they have on their plate, I can see why. It goes a long way to make their job as easy as possible while facilitating what is best for your child. Even if they tell you that you do not need to wash the bottles yourself, it is best to do all you can while you are there. The nurses appreciate it, and it is something you can do that will make you feel like you are helping.

HENRY GOT THE HANG OF DRINKING FROM a bottle after the repositioning and change in bottles. Chuck took to the bottles right away even though he was not able to start until well after Henry. He sucked down everything we gave him and he would want more. He never had a single feeding when he did not finish the entire amount he was given. It was tiring, so some days Henry would finish all that was in his bottle and some days he seemed to finish nothing. It took a long time for him to work up to staying awake for every bottle and finish the entire amount in that bottle. I was trying to learn how to feed him bottles properly but also trying to breastfeed. It made sense that those feeding times for which I was at the hospital were breastfeeding opportunities, but he did not take to nursing and always needed a bottle afterwards. We kept trying, but it was discouraging to realize that he was not getting the hang of it. The lactation consultant said that it was more the exception rather than the rule that micro preemies end up being able to breastfeed. She was very encouraging about continuing to try, but she did not delude me into thinking it was going to be something we would be able to do for sure.

* * * * *

Feeding a preemie or a micro preemie can be much more difficult than you would think. Do not get discouraged. Your nurses can walk you through it and can give tips, but burping and feeding techniques may seem foreign. Henry had to be rotated 180 degrees to burp, which felt very awkward at first. Both boys needed chin support when they were given a bottle. It was hard to figure out how to hold the bottle and also give him some resistance under his chin so that his muscles could work more effectively to suck on the bottle nipple.

* * * * *

The nurses are great at the NICU, but a baby needs feeding 8 times a day and that is a lot. Your nurse probably has additional babies for whom they are caring that may have the same feeding requirements. While they are trained to handle the schedule, the more you can be present for feedings the better. It is more practice for when you are on your own at home.

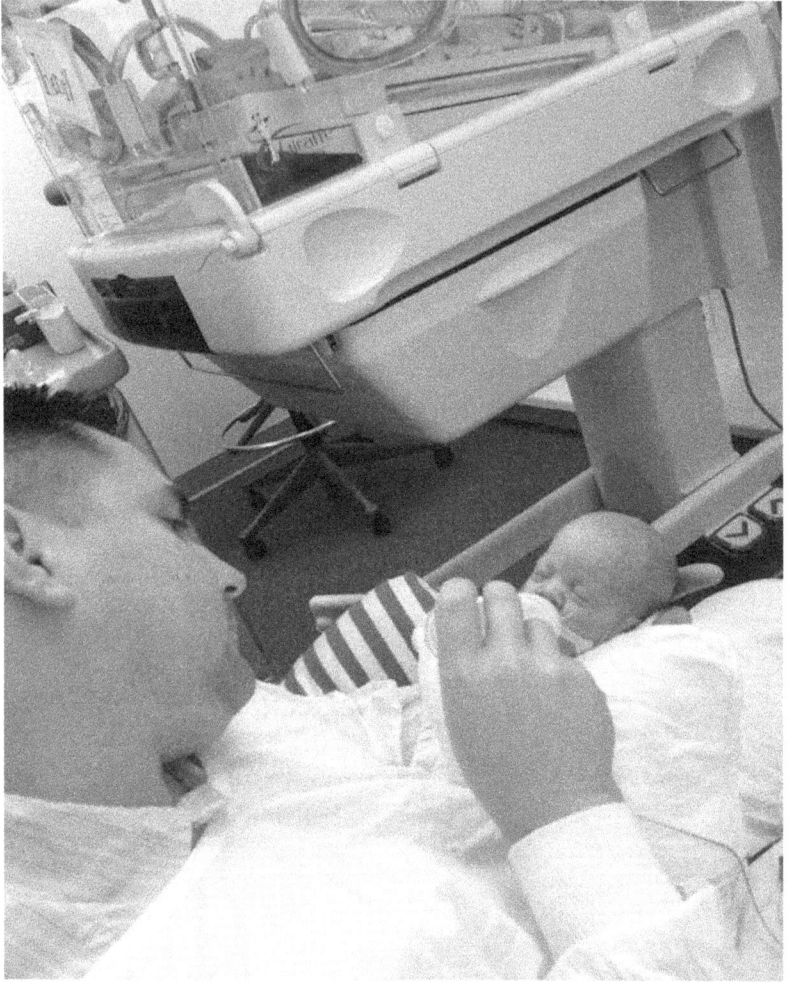

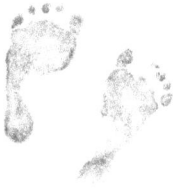

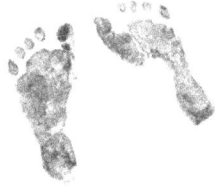

<u>Everyone Cares</u>

WE WERE CONSTANTLY GETTING REMINDERS of how well everyone at the hospital knew our babies because we had been there so long. We would see the Pedi Surg team members walking into or out of the hospital and they would say hello. One of our night nurses had been training another nurse and so had not taken care of the boys for a month, but when she came back to visit them and see how they were doing she brought fleece blankets she had seen at the store and picked up for them. They were perfect, since the NICU is cool at night, and they were great for helping the boys keep their temperatures up in the open cribs. When Chuck's surgeon was in the pod for another baby, he would always stop by to let us know he was just waiting for Chuck's weight to hit the magic number before he could operate for his reversal. The Pedi Surg team always knew exactly how close he was. The receptionists now knew both my husband and me and who our boys were and asked how they were doing when we would sign in to visit every day. It was both reassuring to know so many of the hospital staff were rooting for the boys but also disappointing that they had been in the hospital so long that the staff had all had time to get to know them.

I had joined a Moms of Multiples group in my area the month before the boys had been born. We did not immediately announce their birth to more than very close family and friends, but because my MoMs group had a private Facebook page to which only members had access I felt comfortable after a few days to post an update there. Even though I had only been to a single meeting and did not really know anyone, I let the group know the boys had been born and at which hospital NICU they were. The number of positive messages of support the other moms offered was overwhelming. They asked for updates and let me know they were thinking of us and were available to help with whatever we needed. I ended up being able to meet two of them for lunch around the hospital when they were in the area. I was glad I had that support, especially from other moms who had dealt with the NICU, before we let all of our friends and family know the boys had been born.

* * * * *

Joining my local Moms of Multiples group was one of the best things I did when I was pregnant. I continue to enjoy the monthly meetings, book club, and Facebook page. It is a great place to ask questions since chances are someone has been through what you are now experiencing.

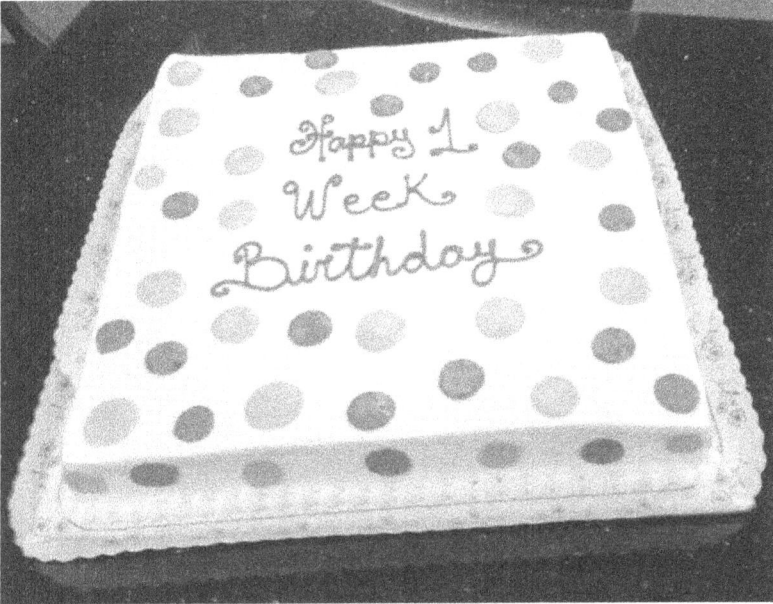

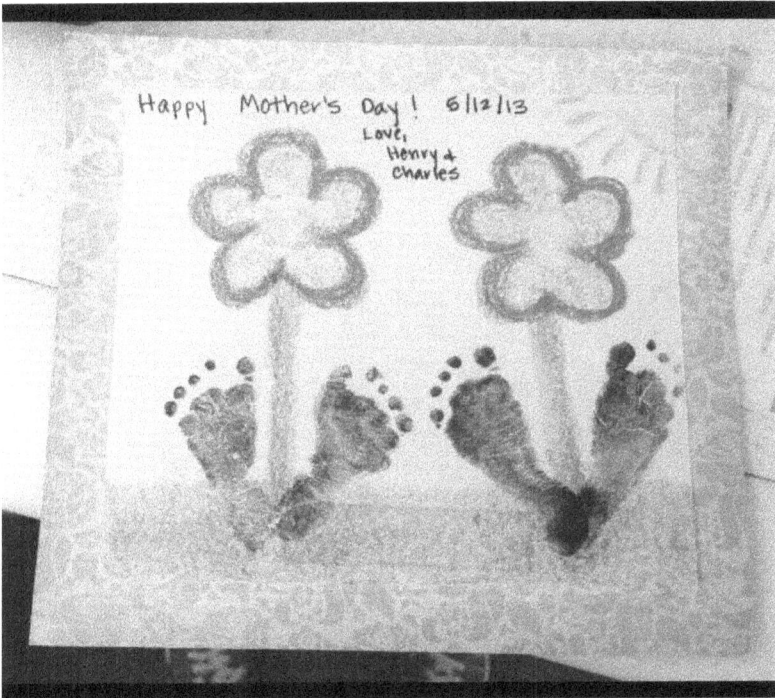

Tiny

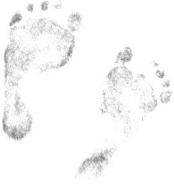

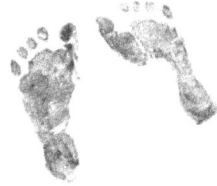

<u>Going Home Tests</u>

BEFORE HENRY COULD GO HOME HE NEEDED to have a hearing test, pass his car seat test, have zero As and Bs for 7 days, and drink all 8 of his bottles a day within 30 minutes for four days in a row. He could use the cannula for bottles because some babies go home still needing that additional oxygen. It was pretty surprising when we heard one morning he had started the 7 day countdown for the first time. It meant we were very close to having him come home. Those last few tests are very important, but they are also fairly inconsequential in the grand scheme of things considering how far the boys had come. Henry's As and Bs clock got reset a few times and he needed a little extra time to get used to finishing all 8 bottles a day without getting tired. He also had a change in what he had been eating. Typically micro preemies cannot gain weight fast enough on breastmilk alone; therefore, it is fortified with additional calories before it is given to the baby. Because I still wanted to try to breastfeed, the nutritionist and Henry's neonatologist decided giving him 3 bottles of higher calorie formula and 5 bottles of breastmilk/nursing attempts would work best. That meant I did not have to fortify all 8 bottle and have zero breastfeeding opportunities. During his 7 day countdown, we started that regime so he had time to get used to it and prove he was still gaining weight before we went home. The goal was to be off of the formula as soon as possible while continuing to gain well on breastmilk alone. The hospital was comfortable starting the process of weaning off the formula and said we could continue it at home with the pediatrician.

* * * * *

Ask lots of questions when your baby is getting ready to come home since you probably will not have such experienced nurses at your disposal after you are home. Since the boys had come so early, we had not yet thought about things like going home outfits, wipes, and simple medications like Tylenol that are important to have at home. Nurses are great for helping you remember what you will need.

* * * * *

Parents of a NICU baby might not have asked for help while their baby was in the hospital, but when they are getting ready to come home, it is a good time to offer things like babysitting a sibling or house cleaning. Bringing home a baby from the NICU can be different than bringing home a full term healthy baby and extra help at that time may be appreciated. For us, meals after the boys got home were much appreciated.

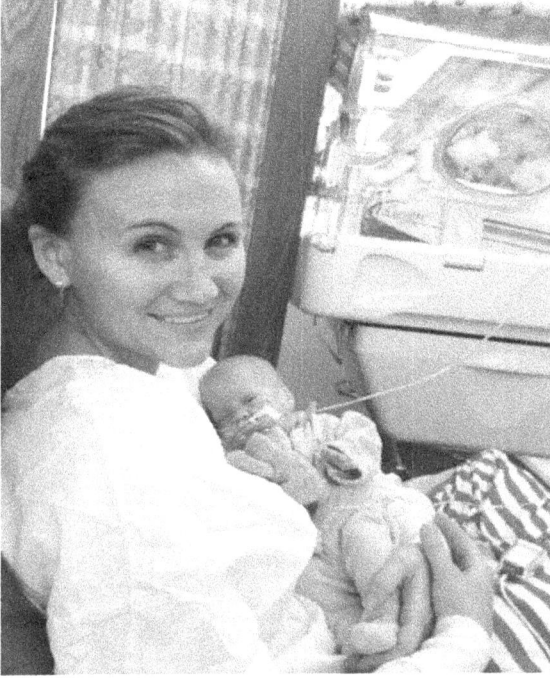

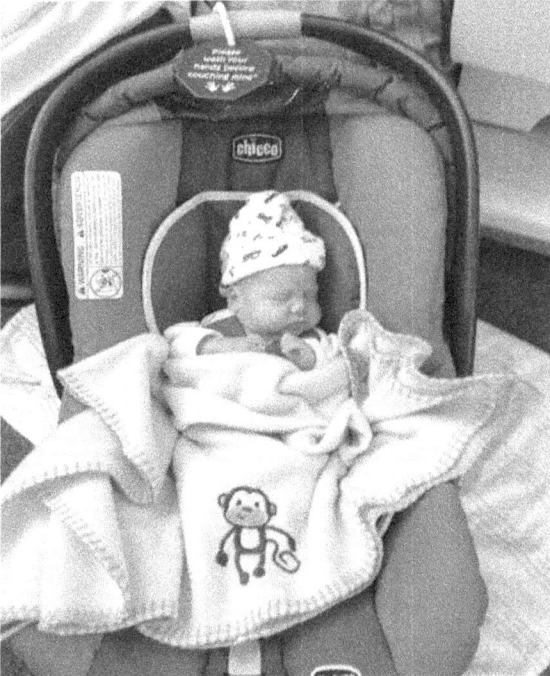

Tiny

I Do Not Have a Pediatrician Yet

AS MUCH OF A PLANNER AS I TYPICALLY AM, I missed out on a couple of things I had wanted to do in the last months of my pregnancy because of how early the boys arrived. I had signed up for a hospital tour (which would have been useless even if we had done it before the boys were born since we ended up at a different hospital), an infant care class (we pretty much learned everything there was to know from the nurses in the NICU, so that turned out okay) and a breastfeeding class (we did end up using the lactation specialists at the hospital for extra help). What we also missed out on was interviewing pediatricians. I did not even know how to go about getting a recommendation for a pediatrician since I did not have any mom friends in the area to ask before the boys were born. Luckily the MoMs group I joined was great at giving recommendations when it got closer to the boys being discharged. I also asked one of our NICU nurses who had a 2 year old. Two of the recommended names were the same, and I started with those two. I called both offices to schedule what they called an "expectant mother" appointment where I could meet with the pediatrician and ask questions.

Both offices had problems trying to schedule me because the first question they asked was the baby's due date. I had to explain our situation and the fact that the boys had already been born. Initially they both told me I could not have an appointment and would have to make a regular appointment when the boys were discharged. I did not accept that because I thought it was ridiculous I could not at least meet with our pediatrician before bringing them my baby since our boys would have a complicated medical history and I was not going to just assume the pediatrician would be a good match for us sight unseen. I had to explain how I did not have two healthy babies sitting at home needing an appointment, but rather I had given birth

16 weeks early and both boys were still in the NICU and I needed to meet with the pediatrician to make sure they were comfortable dealing with the medical history we would have. Both offices had to call me back after talking to supervisors, but thankfully they both figured out how to give me an appointment. I was disappointed I would have to miss two morning visits with the boys, but I was happy I could at least be able to speak with the doctors.

I did not have a clue what questions I should be asking a possible pediatrician. I spent some time online and put together a list of questions along with the list of conditions and diagnoses the boys had on their charts. I was surprised the next day when one of the pediatricians called me from his cell phone on his way home and explained that he had been informed of our situation and with two babies still in the NICU he wanted to save me a visit to the office by having a conversation over the phone. I thought it was extremely thoughtful and we spoke for 20 minutes about how many preemies and micro preemies he had cared for, how familiar and comfortable he was dealing with babies who had been through what the boys had and how familiar he was with things we may be dealing with in the future. By the end of the conversation I was confident and comfortable that he would be a good fit for us and let him know the hospital would call to schedule our first appointments as soon as one of the boys was discharged. I was able to cancel the other appointment I had made and felt good about now having a pediatrician.

* * * * *

If you do not have a pediatrician yet and want to meet with a few before making your decision, you should be able to. Any office which cannot accommodate this request probably is not an office you want to be a part of. It may take a little explaining, but you should be able to speak with pediatricians before you decide who your child will see.

* * * * *

Make a list of conditions and concerns your child has had in the NICU and/or will continue to have upon discharge (your nurses can help with this) and make sure the pediatrician has either dealt with them before or is comfortable dealing with them now. Ask how many babies born as early as yours the pediatrician has within their practice. Additional areas of concern may be breastfeeding, when your child will see a doctor other than your primary pediatrician, how well baby visits work, how same day sick baby visits work, if communication is by text, phone or email, what after-hours care entails, what hospitals and emergency rooms the pediatrician is connected to, what typical waiting times are, and in house versus out of house labs.

* * * * *

We love our pediatrician and I am glad we got the recommendation from our NICU nurses and my MoM's group. If your nurses or friends do not have a suggestion as to where to start looking for a pediatrician, the discharge nurse or social worker should. You will not be discharged without the hospital making your first pediatrician appointment for you, so making sure you have a pediatrician as your baby is getting close to leaving is a must.

Tiny

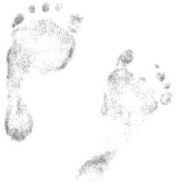

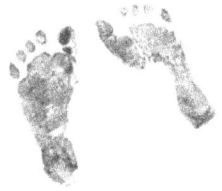

Giving Up the Breastfeeding Dream

I HAD REALLY WANTED TO BREASTFEED MY BOYS. It was something I had actually looked forward to when thinking about having kids. A lot of expectations changed when we had the boys at 24 weeks. I knew initially I had to pump for them, but our nurses were great about always reminding the attending and fellows that I wanted to breastfeed so that we could schedule practice. Henry and I had some success in the hospital; a few times I felt that we had gotten it right and I did not offer him a bottle afterwards because I was sure he was full. But most of the time when I gave a bottle afterwards he took almost as much as if I had not breastfed him first. I tried nipple shields (soft silicone cone-like devices that go over the nipple and can make it easier for a baby to latch) which I hated and did not seem to help much. I also read online that even if the baby learns to breastfeed well using a nipple shield, it can take months to wean them off and become successful breastfeeding without it. Because it had been so important for Chuck to gain weight and because he had been on TPN for so long, we had not even tried to breastfeed at the hospital. We simply wanted him home as soon as possible, and if that meant using bottles then that meant using bottles. All the doctors and nurses were encouraging that once we were home we could ask the pediatrician about trying to breastfeed with him.

Both boys came home taking 8 bottles a day (every 3 hours around the clock), 4 of which were breastmilk and 4 of which were high calorie formula. Regular newborn formula is 20 calories per ounce. I was mixing formula powder at a different ratio with water to make it 24 calories per ounce. The boys needed the extra calories to continue to gain weight as well as they were. Luckily, our pediatrician agreed that the goal was to wean them off the formula as soon as possible and felt having them on just the breastmilk was as important as

I did. At every monthly visit we were able to drop one formula bottle in favor of one breastmilk bottle with both boys. Within no time, they were both only on pumped breastmilk. Initially I would try to nurse Henry before a few of his bottles every day. It continued to be pretty frustrating at home. Most of the time he would drink as much from the bottle that I offered after he trying to nurse as he normally would. I got discouraged. He got frustrated. I was always hot and upset and I was a sweaty anxious mess. It was not fun or enjoyable and it was more time consuming. It was a lot of work for zero pay-off and no progress.

After a few weeks of this, I realized I enjoyed giving Henry bottles much more than I enjoyed our attempts to breastfeed. I decided to stop for one day. For one day I exclusively pumped while I fed him from a bottle and it was such a relief. I felt a little guilty and very disappointed, but it only took one day to realize my breastfeeding dream was dead. I told myself I had a new dream- a pumping dream- and I wanted to make it to at least one year (12 month adjusted, so the boys would actually be 16 months old) before I stopped pumping. That would get us through flu season and hopefully by that time they would be big and strong and ready for real food, so that my stopping pumping would not affect them that much.

I tried to keep in mind that it is great to have goals. Pumping for 16 months is a lofty goal. If you have done that or more, my hat is truly off to you. In reality, I only made it 11 months. I say only because I was disappointed that I could not pump until they "should" have been one year old. That was how long I had originally wanted to breastfeed for, minimum, and I was not able to do it.

Pumping was never a joy, but all of a sudden when I hit month 11, I began to have serious pain when I pumped. It was not mastitis; I knew because I had had that twice already. It just plain hurt. I think it was my body's way of telling me it was done. Pumping is very unnatural and is not fun under the best of circumstances, but to try to continue in constant pain was too much for me. I had read about how to stop breastfeeding or pumping and planned to stop very slowly to try to avoid yet another bout of mastitis. At the beginning of month 11, I began to decrease the amount of each pumping session by 5 minutes every week. I also tried to wait as long as I could between pumping. I had gotten advice that wearing two tight sports bras would help and I did that as well. That made it a lot more comfortable. It took about 5 weeks, but I went from pumping for 25 minutes 5 times a day to not at all. I had already gone through my enormous stash of milk in the freezer so when I was done we gave the boys formula. And I felt guilty about that. I have never heard an argument that breastmilk is not better than formula, and I wanted to give the boys what was best for them. But formula exists for a reason and I tried to remember that the nurses told me there are plenty of smart, happy, wonderful kids who drank formula. I know it to be true, but it took me a while to not wish I had been able to go longer pumping. Eventually I saw the positives of being done.

Once I weaned myself off pumping, I was actually able to hold the boys against my chest without real discomfort for the first time. They may have been a year old, but it was the first time I could comfortably cuddle with them. I do not know what breastfeeding is like. From what I have been told, I have to guess it is better than pumping. My chest was uncomfortable the entire time I was pumping and nothing against it-not a bra, a shirt, a hug, or a baby-felt good. Ever. Getting to snuggle and enjoy it for the first time was something I had not pictured happening when my boys were a year old. Also, being able to shut off all the pumping alarms on my phone and not have to plan the entire day and night around being home for when I was going to pump next was pretty great. It cut down on time during the day I had previously spent washing pumping parts, and it allowed me more sleep at night since I was not feeding the boys and then pumping afterwards. For months before I stopped pumping the boys could drink a bottle faster than the 25 minutes I needed to pump. During the day I was trying to play with them when they were done with their bottle, but I was still pumping. At night I would feed them a bottle and then pump in the dark in their room (since that is where we fed them during the day and where I pumped, that is where the pump lived). It only made sense to put them back to sleep as soon as they were finished with their bottle and not have them sit there in their bouncy chairs and wait for me to finish in the middle of the night. Therefore, when I stopped pumping and only had to feed them a bottle in the middle of the night, I got to go back to sleep as soon as they did. When I finally stopped pumping, it was the first time I was actually looking forward to when the boys were not waking for a bottle in the middle of the night because I could finally see a full night's sleep on the horizon for the first time in about 14 months.

* * * * *

There is nothing wrong with trying and trying again to breastfeed. After a few months of exclusively pumping, I asked the pediatrician if it would be wrong to try again and if he ever thought the boys would get the hang of it. He said we absolutely could try but that the odds were slim they would catch on at this point. He told us there is often a misconception with the term "nipple confusion". He said that it was not that babies were confused between breasts and bottles; it was that once on bottles babies realize that bottles are easier and do not want to go back to the breast. Because the boys had been on bottles so long, it was doubtful they would want to breastfeed, which would be harder for them. There is no rule, however, that says you cannot try. I did try a few times. It was laughable and a complete failure, but at least I would not be left wondering what would have happened if we had tried again.

* * * * *

Pumping is a wonderful thing you can do for your preemie or micro preemie. The fact that your baby is getting breastmilk is the important thing, not how they are getting it. Any breastmilk is good breastmilk. I was lucky I had a great supply and could produce in a day more than or enough of what the boys were eating in a day for 8 whole months. After that their needs surpassed my production and I dipped into my freezer and kept up for another 3 months. I know some moms who would only pump a few ounces a day but kept it up through flu season because they knew how important it was for their small babies. I applaud them. I cannot imagine all the work pumping is for that little of a reward. But any milk is great so do not get discouraged.

*****

There are lots of ways to donate milk if you have abundance. I filled our upright freezer while the boys were in the hospital and needed to get rid of some of the older milk to make room for more before they came home. I was referred to the Mother's Milk Bank of Austin© and was able to donate 400 ounces to them. I could donate milk I had already produced and frozen in traditional breastmilk bags and did not have to use any special containers. When Chuck was discharged from the hospital, I still had 300 ounces in the hospital freezers and no room at home. The lactation department at the hospital was able to take care of it for me and get it to the milk bank.

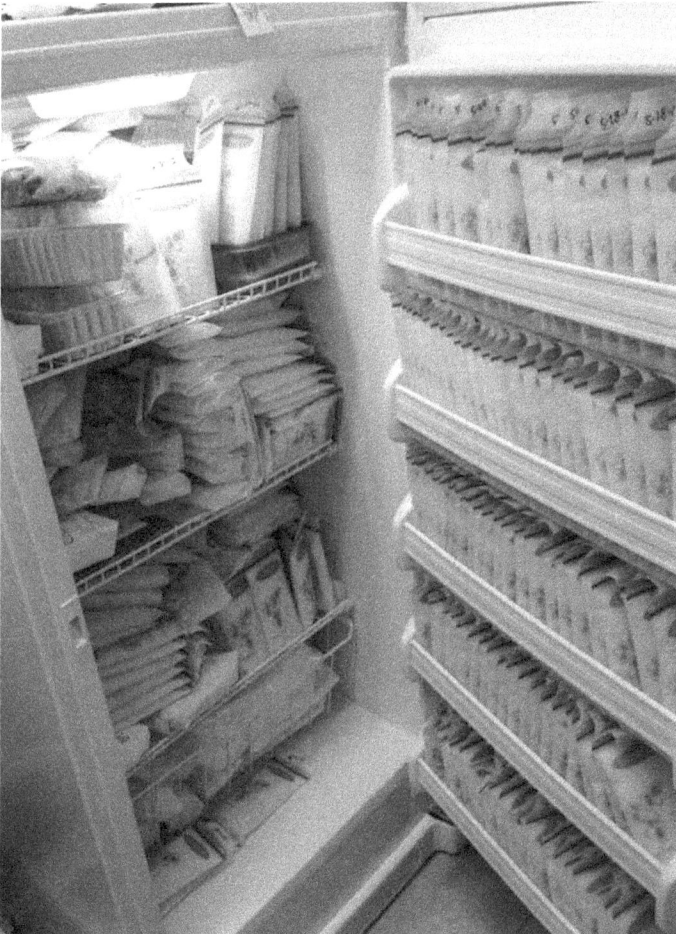

Tiny

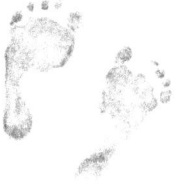

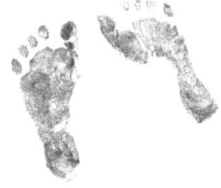

One In and One Out

AS FALL BEGAN, HENRY PASSED HIS CAR SEAT test, had no As and Bs, and continued to finish all his bottles in the allotted time. He was ready to come home. After 105 days in the NICU, and at a hefty 5 pounds, 14.5 ounces he was officially discharged. It was incredibly exciting and also very sad because we had to leave behind Chuck. My husband took the day off and we arrived in the morning with celebratory doughnuts for everyone, a going home onesie that read "2013 NICU Grad," and our first ever packed diaper bag. The nurses loaded us down with everything that was in his crib (open wipes containers, diapers, diaper cream, nose aspirators, scissors, thermometer, extra formula-basically anything not needing to immediately be thrown away that we could possibly use we were given). As soon as rounds were over, his information from the previous 24 hours was entered into the computer and his paperwork was readied. We then took off his leads, dressed him, and signed his discharge paperwork. We got a few copies of his paperwork, which summarized his time in the NICU, and were given a list of follow up appointments that had been made for us. We would see the pediatrician in a few days, I would have to bring him back downtown for a follow up for his studies and to see the endocrine team in two weeks, and we would see the ophthalmologist when he turned one. It was a short list of appointments for someone who had been in the NICU for so long.

* * * * *

Put a copy of your discharge paperwork in a zip top bag and leave it in your diaper bag. That way, anytime you need to see anyone in the medical profession outside the hospital that discharged your baby they can quickly and efficiently read a summary of your baby's medical history. If you are ever in an ER out of town, it may be quite difficult for you to remember everything important for the medical team to know. With the discharge summary in your diaper bag anytime you are out of your house, you have the medical history with you.

IT WAS VERY DIFFICULT TO BE HAPPY THAT WE were taking Henry home because we had to leave Chuck at the hospital. We knew this would change how often we could visit Chuck since Henry would not be allowed back in the NICU and one of us would need to stay home with him at all times. We had decided one of us would visit every night so that Chuck would not go a single day without a parent. My schedule of pumping every 3 hours and trying to breastfeed Henry a few times a day complicated visiting Chuck even further. We kept the boys on the same 3 hour feeding schedule, so once my husband came home from work I could pump and immediately leave for the hospital. Meanwhile at home, my husband would continue Henry's 3 hour schedule with pumped milk from the freezer or the formula since he was not on all breastmilk yet. I tried to pump right before I left the hospital after visiting with Chuck or I would have to pump as soon as I got home. I would get home close to 11 pm and would take over waking and feeding Henry. It was tough to leave the hospital with Chuck there, but it was also difficult to be away from Henry at home. I had not slept more than about an hour and 45 minutes at a time since the day Henry was born, which added to the chaos.

We had hoped Chuck would have his reanastimosis surgery to reconnect his intestines and put everything back in his abdomen before Henry came home because that would have allowed both my husband and I to stay at the Ronald McDonald House™ room overnight and be at the hospital for the surgery while both boys were still in the NICU. However, since Chuck had not met the weight requirement by the time Henry was ready to come home, the surgery did not happen. As it turned out, Chuck hit the magic number 5 days after Henry was discharged. My husband took the day off work to be there for his early morning surgery. He stayed over in the Ronald McDonald House™ room the night before since the surgery was the first scheduled the following morning and he needed to begin signing paperwork at 6 am. I could not think about anything else except how Chuck was doing, but I was glad I was not the one there with him because that would have made me more nervous.

My husband and I spoke to one of Chuck's nurses about him getting an epidural for his surgery. He would have to be put under general anesthesia and on a ventilator for the surgery. An epidural was not required, and he would have to have general anesthesia regardless, but his surgeon explained it might help wean him off the vent sooner because his pain control could be through the epidural and not morphine. However, it also might not help him with the vent and was an additional risk on top of the procedure. I was worried about adding something else to the surgery that was not completely necessary. Pediatric anesthesiologists, even those at specialized children's hospitals like ours, simply do not have the opportunity to do many epidurals on babies as small as ours. On one hand, I trusted the surgeon completely and he was recommending the epidural, but on the other hand, I trusted Chuck's nurse completely and she was not. My husband did not feel strongly either way so it was basically up to me to decide. I felt strongly that I did not want him to have it. My husband called the morning of the surgery after speaking to the surgeon to give me one more opportunity to consent to the epidural. I was very stressed out about making the decision, but I said I did not want him to have it.

Chuck did amazingly well during his surgery. His surgeon did not have to remove additional bowel, which was great, and gave every indication that Chuck should heal with no lasting complications. Although it was his third surgery, it was the first time Chuck went downstairs to the operating room with the transport team instead of being operated on in the NICU because he was big and healthy enough to do so. He came back to his pod with the transport team and into an open warmer instead of an incubator so they could keep him only diapered in order to watch his incision carefully for infection for the next few days. When he got back to the NICU, my husband saw Chuck without his ostomy bag for the first time since he was 4 days old and immediately texted me the photo. I sent it to his nurses who were not working that day for them to see he did well and that he was out of surgery.

The next steps for Chuck were pain management and extubation. He needed morphine for the first few days, but he could not be weaned off the vent while on morphine because it suppressed his desire to breathe well enough on his own. It was going to be a bit of a tightrope walk to give him morphine long enough to keep him pain-free but also get him off as soon as possible so he could get off the vent. We were both surprised to see the ostomy hole had been left open and not closed with stitches. His incision from the first surgery had been reopened and lengthened (from his belly button, which was not really a belly button anymore, almost all the way to the middle of his right side), so that the bowel could be run again to make sure everything was healthy and then that larger incision line was stitched up. The ostomy hole where his two intestine ends had protruded out, however, was not closed. His wound was bright red in color, but it looked healthy, as though a nickel-sized hole had been cut out of his skin with a cookie cutter.

It was my turn to visit the night after the surgery. When Pedi Surg came by to look at him and change his dressing, they spoke with me. They said he had done as they had hoped he would during surgery and explained that they had left the ostomy open because of how low on his torso it was, how close to the other incision it was, and because the risk of infection from fecal matter was too great to chance closing the wound and not seeing an infection for a period of time. Leaving it open allowed for it to heal naturally and for it to be monitored much more closely for infection. We were all shocked how quickly it closed. At first it was covered with some iodinated strips and gauze to prevent his diaper rubbing against it. After a week it was healed over with a scab and he did not need the iodinated strips anymore and we put gauze between his skin and his diaper. We continued to cover it with gauze at home until we were told by the pediatrician he had healed enough to stop.

While Chuck was recovering from surgery, Henry had his first pediatrician appointment. He had gained 6 ounces in the 5 days since he left the hospital and his pediatrician was pleased. We were able to drop one of his formula bottles a day and replace it with breastmilk. One week after that we were able to drop the last formula bottle so he was entirely on breastmilk. The pediatrician gave us a chart listing typical milestones for the first 12 months of a baby's life and asked us to write down the month each baby completed each milestone to make sure they were progressing normally.

* * * * *

Babies born significantly before their due date are usually given more time to catch up to their peers in terms of milestones before they are considered delayed. The term "adjusted age" refers to how old the baby would be if they had been born full term. Since our boys were 16 weeks early, when Henry came home he was 5 months old, 1 month adjusted. We were not excepting him to do all the things a full term 5 month old could. Keeping track of the boys' milestones for the first two years let us see how close they were to catching up to their full term peers.

CHUCK'S BREATHING CONTINUED TO IMPROVE and his vent was weaned down slowly in hopes of getting off as soon as possible after the morphine was taken away. It took 6 days for him to finally poop after surgery, and we were all very excited because that indicated his bowels were working as they should. After a few days the drain into his belly came out and, although he could not be fed except through his OG tube until he was off the vent, he was able to start breastmilk again through the tube into his belly. The orange color to his skin started to go away as the TPN was lowered and the breastmilk was increased. His nurses were beginning to notice him breathing faster than the vent, which was a good sign that he was getting ready to be extubated. We had been hoping he would be able to come off the vent in 48 hours, but he was just beginning to show signs that he was ready on day 5 after surgery. That was disappointing, especially since I felt that it had been my decision to not have the epidural that could have possibly made it easier for him to come off the vent. Every day he went beyond the first 48 hours, I questioned my decision and felt very guilty that perhaps I had made the wrong one. His neonatologist was positive he was working at his own pace and did not question my decision, but it was hard not to second guess myself anyway.

* * * * *

Make sure you think realistically about decisions you are making and try not to feel guilty if something does not go according to your plan. I made decisions with the best available information and after having talked to doctors, nurses, and surgeons. If something you are advocating for is way off base, your baby's medical team will surely tell you so. However, no one can see the future and promise you things will go well if you do one thing or another. While everyone is well trained, remember that they are super specialized advocates. These babies are very fragile and things can get much worse or much better at the drop of a hat. Sometimes you need to remember that you made the best decision you could have at the time and move forward.

AFTER HENRY CAME HOME WE DECIDED TO ASK my parents to fly in a few days after Chuck's surgery in case I wanted to or needed to be at the hospital with Chuck as he recovered. That would allow my parents to stay at home with Henry while I was downtown at the hospital. I was glad we had made that decision because the day after Chuck was finally extubated he had a particularly bad day. When I called first thing in the morning to check on him his nurse said if I was at all able, she would like me to come down and hold him to try to calm him down. I would not have been able to do that if my parents had not been at my house to watch Henry. Some changes had occurred in Chuck's pod, and there was more activity and more noise than typical. He did not seem to like the changes and was agitated. I drove down immediately and arrived as his nurse was getting ready to give him some blood. His CBC levels the day before had been slightly concerning and the team had tried to wait a day to see whether he could recover or if he needed some blood. His vitals showed he needed the blood.

Babies do not make their own blood before a certain gestational age; therefore, both boys had received blood to replace what had been drawn for tests before they could make more on their own. Chuck was past this point by now, but after surgery it was not uncommon that he would need a little as his body recovered. I put on a gown and held him while the nurse hooked up the drip and he calmed down. Even as experienced as she was, she accidentally got blood all over Chuck and me. I texted my husband a photo of the "blood bath" and he laughed. The blood almost instantly perked Chuck up and things began to turn around from that point. His blood gasses began to get better because the more blood he had in his system the more oxygen could be circulated. Over the next day his team continued to increase the amount of milk and decrease the amount of TPN. When he reached full feeds of milk, he did not need the TPN anymore and he was finally able to have his PICC line removed. He was also gaining weight steadily, which was another great sign his body was able to absorb everything it needed and his intestines were working correctly.

* * * * *

Nurses and nurse practitioners can call you after rounds to let you know if changes were made or what was discussed. After Chuck's surgery we were only able to visit at night, except for the week my parents were in town, which meant missing rounds every week day. My husband and I made a point to make the rounds on weekends, but that is not usually when major changes are made. If nurses or nurse practitioners do not call (some did and some did not), you can always call and ask for an update. I tried not to call until I was sure rounds were over so that I was not calling a million times and asking for information that was not available yet.

ITTOOKALITTLE OVER TWO WEEKS FOR CHUCK to go from getting all his feeds through his OG tube to starting bottles, to stopping the TPN and getting his PICC line out, to passing his hearing and car seat tests. He failed his hearing test a grand total of 4 times before finally passing it, but the nurses were great about letting us know why they felt he was failing and that it was not him but the incubator or the ventilator that was disallowing the machine from getting an accurate read.

* * * * *

Do not worry needlessly about failed tests without asking your nurses and doctors. Every baby's initial blood screen after birth is sent to state and national databases, and I was warned many times that I would be receiving letters about the boys' not meeting standards for liver function, among other things. It is totally normal for very premature babies to fail lots of tests, only to retake them at or around the appropriate adjusted age and pass.

AFTER HE WAS FINALLY EXTUBATED AFTER surgery, Chuck had many ups and down with trying to come off the cannula. He could not go from being on the vent to having no support, so he went onto the cannula the day after he was extubated. It took a few days for him to master breathing without any support. He had been on 21% oxygen (the same as room air) on his cannula for an entire day when, during rounds, one of his nurses gave him a bottle. The team saw him sitting on her lap looking at all of them as they rounded on all the babies. His breathing was so impressive without the cannula that it was taken away except for during bottle feedings if his breathing dipped and he required it. They also decided to try 4 bottles of breastmilk and 4 bottles of 24 calorie formula every 24 hours, the same as Henry had gone home on. However, after a few days, the night nurses were still having trouble keeping his oxygen where it needed to be overnight. He seemed to need the cannula at night, but during the day he would be taken off again and his oxygen would be fine.

* * * * *

It is hard when it seems like your baby is so close to going home but is still experiencing two steps forward and one step back. I tried to keep in mind how far we had come and realize that the things Chuck was struggling with were so inconsequential in the grand scheme of all he had accomplished thus far. We tried not to get antsy about when Chuck would be able to come home and give him the time he needed to master the last few things before coming home.

FINALLY, AFTER NUMEROUS NIGHTS ON A CANNULA and days without, the team decided that they would write an order for him to go home with a cannula and oxygen monitor for bottle feeds and whenever else we felt we needed it. Since that was the only thing keeping him in the NICU, they felt confident he could come home. It would be up to us to try to keep the oxygen settings as low as possible to allow him to work to come off needing it and also to not overload him on oxygen. It was disappointing to hear he would come home with monitors, but we were glad it did not mean he needed to stay in the hospital only to figure out the breathing situation. We were also pleasantly surprised to hear that his ophthalmologist had decided his vision was stable enough that he did not need to see her again until his first birthday. With all of those last issues ironed out, he was officially ready to come home. It was a very sleepless night the night before we were to go and pick him up because I was very worried some other issue would come up and prevent us from taking him home. I called the morning he was to be discharged and held my breath as I asked his nurse how the night had gone and whether he could still be discharged. I let out a long sigh of relief when she said he had had a great night and was waiting for us. After a tearful goodbye our nurse took a photo of our fully discharged boys and us and we left the hospital as a family of four for the first time, 134 days after the boys were born.

* * * * *

It was such a relief to be home but also a little nerve wracking that it was the first time we were fully on our own with 'newborns'. It took a few hours but we eased into our 3 hour feed routine and slowly found our rhythm.

* * * * *

Friends and family are probably nearly as excited as you are that your NICU baby has come home. Some parents want everyone over to share in the joy, but others may want some time alone with their baby to get into their groove. We were lucky that our friends and family respected our need to be a family of four for a little while before inviting them over to visit. We knew there would be lots of time to visit in the future, but for a week we wanted to enjoy finally being a family of four at home by ourselves and find our routine with the boys.

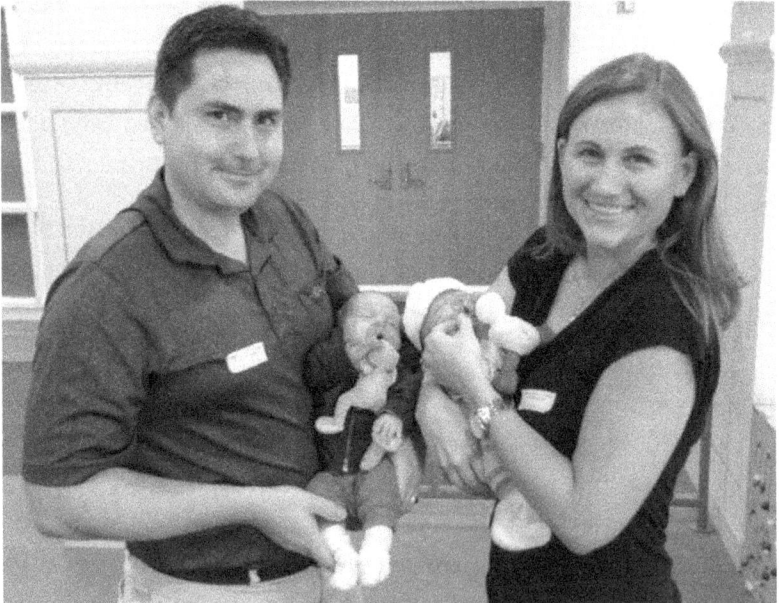

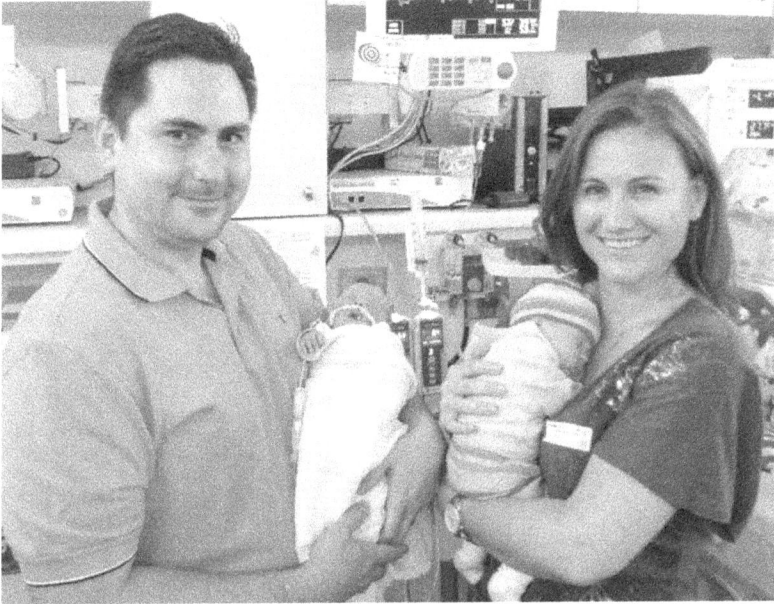

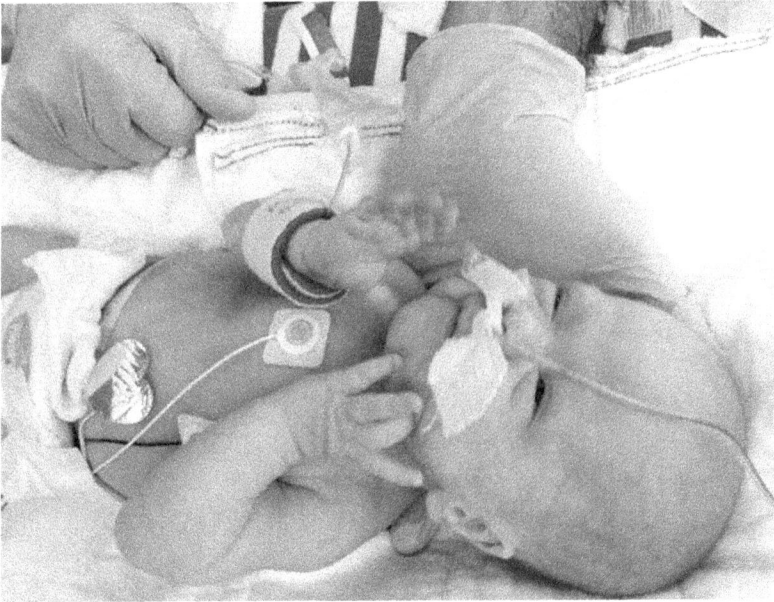

Tiny

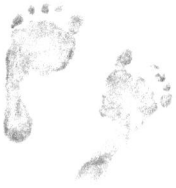

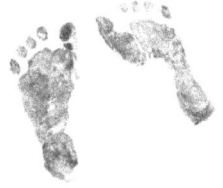

Bringing Home Machines

MANY BABIES COME HOME FROM THE NICU on monitors or with other medical devices. We were lucky that Henry did not need to come home on any monitors. Chuck was still having trouble keeping his oxygen saturation up during his feeds, but otherwise he had mastered everything he needed to in order to be discharged. Therefore, he came home with a pulse ox monitor and oxygen tanks/equipment that we used while we fed him. I was nervous about this at first, but all the nurses assured me it was common and he would hopefully outgrow the need soon. Before he was discharged, the medical supply company came to our house to show us the equipment and teach us to use it. It was more equipment than I expected. Our office-now the feeding room-became home to 1 portable O2 monitor, 2 large boxy machines that filled oxygen tanks, 1 large oxygen tank, one small portable tank and a box filled with extra cannulas.

As it turned out, we were very glad to have the equipment because we noticed Chuck's oxygen saturation drop fairly significantly a few weeks later when he got his second round of immunizations. Immunizations can cause a baby to act as though they are fighting off a virus (exactly what the shot is designed to do as the baby is making their own antibodies) and cause them to feel crummy and work harder than normal. It was very important the boys get all their immunizations quickly and on schedule because their tiny bodies and weak lungs would not be able to effectively or easily fight off the real viruses. We were warned they would likely end up back in the hospital if they got sick. Because we had the O2 monitor, we noticed Chuck was requiring more oxygen and we were able to speak with his pediatrician who told us to use additional oxygen at our discretion until he seemed to recover. For a few days he was doing fine while he was awake, but he continued to sat poorly (his oxygen saturation was low) while he was sleeping on his back for naps and overnight. We spoke with the team again and decided we would use the oxygen at night until he satted better, and then we could use the monitor without the oxygen to test him and make sure he was okay and no longer need the monitor. In the meantime, he was doing great while drinking bottles, so after a month he was off oxygen to eat and only on it while he slept on his back.

A few weeks of Chuck being on oxygen for naps and overnight and I discovered he satted great while sleeping on his tummy so I started napping the boys during the day on their tummies on the couch. We were not comfortable having them sleep that way at night when we were not watching them, because stomach sleeping can increase the risk of SIDS and our boys were already at a higher risk for SIDS due to their prematurity. During the day I could continue to use the oxygen monitor and be physically present while they napped; therefore, I felt confident they were sleeping well and was reassured Chuck was getting enough oxygen. This certainly limited what I was able to get done around the house during the day since I needed to hang around the couch, but it gave Chuck a break from his cannula and I felt as though it was a step in the right direction to eventually being done with oxygen altogether.

When Chuck first came home and only needed the cannula to give him a bottle, we could usually keep it in place on his face fairly well without any tape. While he was sleeping, however, he wanted to turn his head and get the cannula off his face and it was impossible to keep it where it needed to be. When we realized he needed it every night to sleep, one of our nurses brought us a 'cannula kit' with some tegaderm™ and duoDERM® so that we could put protective tape on his cheeks and then additional tape to keep the cannula secure and leave it there all day when we connected and disconnected the tube from the oxygen. The tape worked great while he required oxygen much of the day, but he was really getting sick of it being on his face so giving him a break during naps was nice. It felt as though he was on oxygen forever. Looking back to the day he came home, we knew he was needing less and less help (luckily he only ever needed 1/8 at his highest, which is not much at all). We knew there was a light at the end of the tunnel, but it felt as though it was taking forever to get to it. Finally after only a few months he was satting well enough during the night and naps that he no longer needed oxygen altogether.

* * * * *

You can call your local fire department to let them know if you are using oxygen in your home. You can also let them know when you are finished using it. Our fire department told me that all ambulances were equipped with oxygen and infant masks, but those that would service your home may not be. They were pleased that I had let them know Chuck's situation and put a note by our address, so that if we ever called them they would know before they walked in the door, what the problem might be and they could be more prepared.

* * * * *

Monitors can seem very intimidating at first, but you will quickly get the hang of using them and it will become second nature. You can always call the home health company and ask questions. At one point the small portable oxygen tank we were using full time burst its O ring. I was able to speak with a technician after regular business hours and receive replacement parts the next day. They are there to help you with equipment and I found our company very responsive.

* * * * *

Friends and family may be very unfamiliar with monitors. It may feel like you are a broken record having to explain again and again what the device does, why it is needed and why you cannot get rid of it yet. If friends and family are present to help and do not understand the devices, it may be more helpful to give them another job to do with which they are more comfortable that does not directly involve feeding or holding the baby.

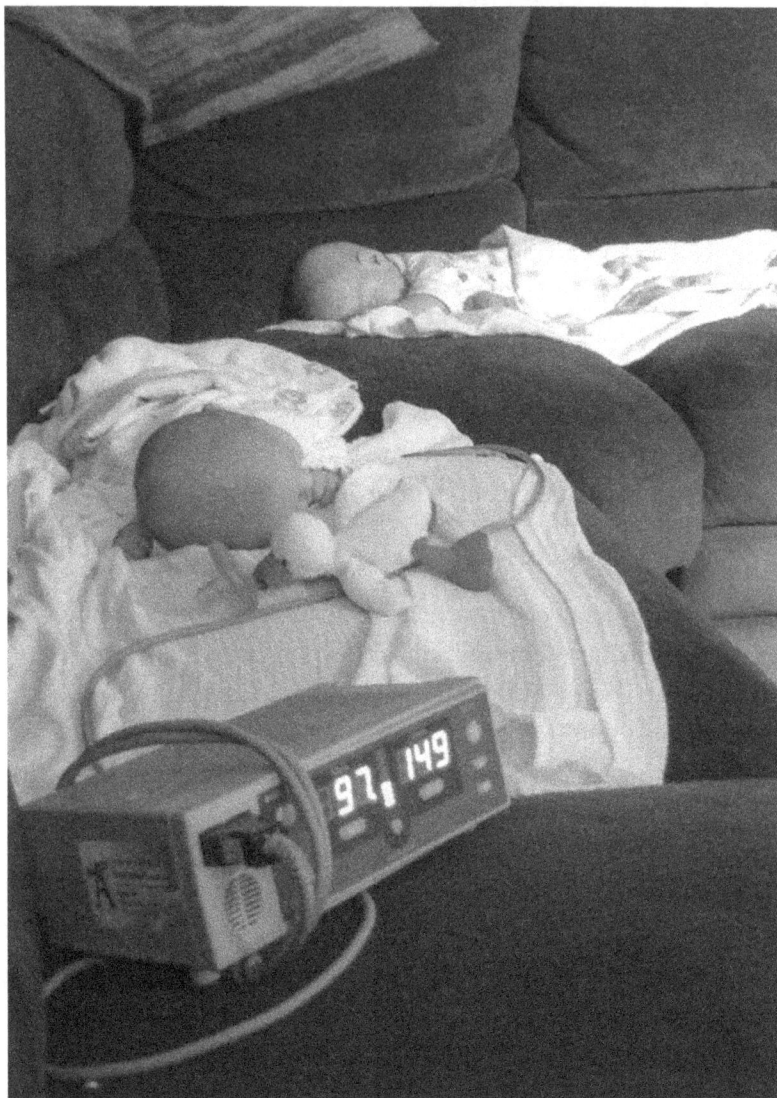

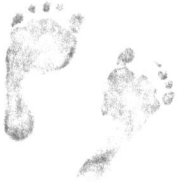

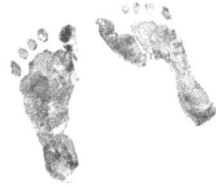

<u>Germs</u>

I HAD NEVER GOTTEN A FLU SHOT BEFORE I was pregnant because I had never had the flu and felt those with a healthy immune system did not need it. After the boys were born, we became very aware of the flu, Pertussis, Respiratory Syncytial Virus (RSV) and germs in general. Neither my husband nor I were big germ-a-phobes, and neither of us had been sick often before the boys were born. However, now we were super vigilant about germs. We were both due for the Pertussis vaccine and we got a dose the day I was discharged. The boys, both due to their prematurity in general and their chronic lung disease from being on the vents, were extremely at risk for catching anything. Not only would the flu or Pertussis make them extremely ill, more ill than a healthy full term baby, it would likely put them back in the hospital. We realized that everyone the boys came into contact with who had not been vaccinated for these diseases increased their risk for ending up back in the hospital.

Both boys were discharged right at the beginning of flu season; therefore, we were advised to not take them in public and not have visitors who felt ill or were unvaccinated until flu season was over. Flu season, in our part of the country, stretches from August until April. It was a bit daunting to think we would be inside for 9 months, but we were determined not to let the boys get sick unnecessarily and absolutely did not want them to end up back in the hospital. We asked any family members who would be visiting at Thanksgiving and Christmas to get both the flu vaccine and the Pertussis vaccine. Luckily all our friends and family completely understood the risks of the boys getting sick and all made sure their vaccines were up to date.

* * * * *

Our NICU provided immunizations (Pertussis, flu) for free to family members and those who would be in contact with the babies when they went home. Make sure you take advantage of this if you or a family member is due.

* * * * *

Friends and family can help limit the spreading of germs by practicing vigilant hand washing and making sure they stay away if they feel ill. One of our nurses told us that even if someone says their congestion is due to allergies, do not believe them! You do not want anyone who could be sick in contact with a baby who has been recently discharged from the NICU. Sure enough, one of our visitors called ahead to say she had allergies but because of what our nurse had told me I asked to reschedule the visit. A week later she said she and her daughter had both actually had the flu. No one wants to put your babies at risk, but we subscribed to the "better safe than sorry" policy and were thankful we had.

WE WERE ADVISED BY OUR NEONATOLOGISTS, as well as our nurses and later by our pediatrician, that the boys' first and second flu seasons would be fairly critical to their overall health. Basically, no one wanted them to leave the house and be in public during their first flu season. The boys would be getting flu shots, Pertussis vaccines, and also RSV prevention shots (given monthly and incredibly expensive/hard to qualify for). None of that was an absolute guarantee that they would not pick up a virus. Getting sick for them was entirely different than a full term baby getting sick. The vaccines lessened the chances they would get sick, and would decrease the severity if they did get sick, but even a minor virus would be a very big deal for our boys, which is why we were trying to avoid everything. We were committed to doing our best to get through flu season without them landing back in the hospital. They had plenty of time to build up an arsenal of antibodies to viruses later in life when they were bigger and stronger. Their very first flu season was not the ideal time to begin that.

Breastfeeding and pumping were a good start to helping them build a healthy immune system since breastmilk carries antibodies. Our nurses told us to buy a million liquid hand sanitizer pumps and spread them all over the house. My husband could use some upon returning from work, I could do the same if I went out while he was home with the boys, and any visitors were asked to wash their hands as soon as they entered the house and to sanitize in between holding each baby. They also cautioned us to only invite close friends and family over and making sure everyone felt well before they came over. We took the boys to the pediatrician once a month for their RSV shot and weigh in and to any other medical appointments that were necessary, but other than that the boys literally did not leave the house from September to March.

We did not even begin walks around the neighborhood until February, because Chuck's oxygen and paraphernalia was too cumbersome. We were also incredibly careful when we took them to medical appointments to cover their car seats completely, so that no one was tempted to reach over and touch them. I purchased signs that hung from their car seat handles that said "Wash your hands before touching mine" to further warn people off. All those things working in concert helped the boys avoid the flu and RSV during one of our region's highest seasons. We were proud all our work had paid off.

* * * * *

Do not apologize for trying to keep your baby healthy even if it means backing out of family gatherings, events in public, or asking someone to reschedule a visit if they are not feeling 100% well. The last thing you need to do is put your baby at risk. Some people thought we were crazy for not bringing the boys anywhere and that for the first 11 months of their lives they literally had not been anywhere but the NICU, our home, and the pediatrician. Most people are not aware of how susceptible preemies and micro preemies are to illness; do not feel you have to explain yourself. I caught myself apologizing for asking family members to get their flu shots before they came to visit that first year. I do not feel that way anymore. It is my number one job to protect my kids, and right now, that is what they need to stay healthy. So many of my friends' healthy full term babies got RSV during the boys' first flu season that I felt validated about all the measures we took to keep them healthy.

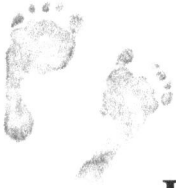

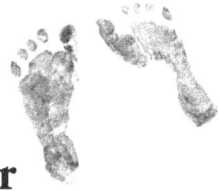

Finally Home Together

IT WAS VERY SURREAL TO BE HOME AS A FAMILY of four for the first time. The boys were over 4 months old when both of them were finally home, but they were actually only a few weeks past their due date. My husband had saved a week of vacation to use when both boys came home so we could be together. After spending our first weekend feeding, pumping, and changing the boys, we got into our routine.

Initially my goal was to pump and feed the boys at the same time every 3 hours, but at first I could not do both. We had brought Henry home feeding him on his side, but by the time Chuck came home he was big enough to drink a bottle that was held for him sitting upright in a bouncy chair. I had envisioned feeding both boys in bouncy chairs while facing them and pumping at the same time. The day before my husband went back to work I attempted this for practice and realized it was impossible for me. Instead, I would feed one while I pumped and then immediately wake the other and feed him while the first had a little play time or went right back to sleep. When the boys first came home we were waking them every 3 hours because they would not wake frequently enough on their own to eat as many calories as they needed every day. After they were fed and burped, I would try to get in some tummy time or would hold them before they fell asleep again. The only difference between the day and night was that at night they fell right back to sleep in their chairs after every bottle. At night after I was done pumping, putting the milk away, and cleaning all the pumping supplies, I would carry two sleeping bundles back to the mini crib in our room and put them down on their backs. Since we were on the 3 hour schedule, I would wake them up about an hour and a half later and do it all again. Chuck's oxygen complicated things a little. Since he needed it to sleep and eat initially, I had to carry his tank with me into the office from the bedroom and then back again, which made for many trips every time I had to feed them.

* * * * *

Do not be afraid to change up the routine and try something new. I thought I could feed the boys and pump at the same time, but I did a trial before my husband went back to work and it was way too stressful. I knew it would take longer to feed one and then the other, but initially it was all I could handle. There is no right way to do things, so ask for suggestions or try other things until you figure out what works best.

* * * * *

If you can buy a few sets of pumping equipment or a ton of bottles, you can wait until the end of the day to wash most things in the dishwasher and avoid hand washing things throughout the day. I had two sets of pumping equipment since I had accidentally left what I needed at home the morning I dashed down for Chuck's unexpected surgery and had to buy a second set at the hospital. It turned out I was grateful to have the second set because I could leave one set in my bag and one set at home while the boys were still in the NICU. When the boys were both home, I then only had to wash my pumping things every other feeding because I had the two sets. We only had enough bottles to get through one day exactly so I always washed bottles after every feeding.

* * * * *

Dish washing gloves became necessary at home because my hands got raw from all the washing.

AFTER OUR FIRST WEEKEND HOME WE HAD a photographer friend come to the house to take some photos since I had been waiting to send out birth announcements until we were home. She and I had been emailing throughout the boys' NICU stay to try to coordinate when she could visit after they came home and how photos would work. Since we were way beyond the typical new-born "cute, squishy pose-able" stage, I told her I simply wanted some nice photos and did not care what the poses were. She is a labor and delivery nurse and has her own twin boys so we could not have asked for a more understanding photographer. She got exactly the shot I envisioned for the boys' birth announcement and some other great photos of us as a family as well. Even our dog got to be involved and it all went as smoothly as it could have. I was excited, after 5 months, to be able to send out a happy birth announcement.

* * * * *

We sent birth announcements to our IVF office and my OB/GYN office as well as to friends and family. Doctors are very happy to hear news that your story had a happy ending if they are aware you went into labor prematurely and your baby needed NICU time.

AFTER A FEW WEEKS AT HOME, THE BOYS started making some sounds and became interested in play gyms and mirrors above their heads. They also both smiled within the first few weeks home. They were definitely beginning to show us their person-alities. By this point I had been pumping every 3 hours around the clock for about 5 months. While the boys were in the NICU, it took me about 30 minutes to pump and take care of the milk so that I could go back to sleep for about two-and-a-half hours. Once the boys came home, it took me about 25 minutes to wake, change, feed one and pump, another 25 minutes to wake, change and feed the other, and then 5 minutes to take care of bottles, pumping equipment and milk. It took a solid hour between my alarm going off and putting the boys back in bed and climbing in myself. If absolutely nothing went wrong and the boys fell asleep immediately and so did I, I could sleep for two hours before my alarm went off again. Two hours a few times overnight before waking for the day between 5 and 6 am is not much sleep, especially when it is preceded by months of two and a half hours of sleep at a time.

Luckily, I have always done okay without a lot of sleep; there-fore, at the time it did not seem too bad. Once my husband went back to work after his week home, I was the only one to take care of the boys during the day and did the midnight to morning shift, so every time the alarm went off to wake and feed them, I needed to do it. With no real alternative, it made the lack of sleep easier to tolerate.

* * * * *

Friends and family, unless they have had multiples, probably do not know how difficult dealing with multiple newborns is. They might think the babies are somehow easier to handle because they may be "old" from having spent days or months in the NICU. However, that does not really make things any easier. Especially if babies were born early, parents are going to be more tired when their baby finally comes home because they have already dealt with the stress and sleep deprivation for days or months before even beginning their at-home parenting.

* * * * *

When a baby is discharged from the NICU, it is a great time to offer to bring a meal, come do laundry, iron, clean, or pick up groceries for parents. Even though the babies may seem older, they are most likely not allowed to sleep for very long stretches at a time. Even just an adult conversation is sometimes nice.

* * * * *

Remember not to make more work for the parents if you are visiting a recently discharged NICU baby (e.g., do not leave your drinks or coffee cups around the house when you visit, ask to stay for a meal you were not invited for or leave your personal belongings where the parents have to clean them up. If you are staying overnight, do not leave your clothing and personal items everywhere. Offer to strip beds or do laundry before you leave). Taking care of a newborn is time consuming! Do not ask the parent of twins, recently home from the hospital, to babysit your own children in addition to their own, cook you a meal when you are visiting, or add to their workload in any way.

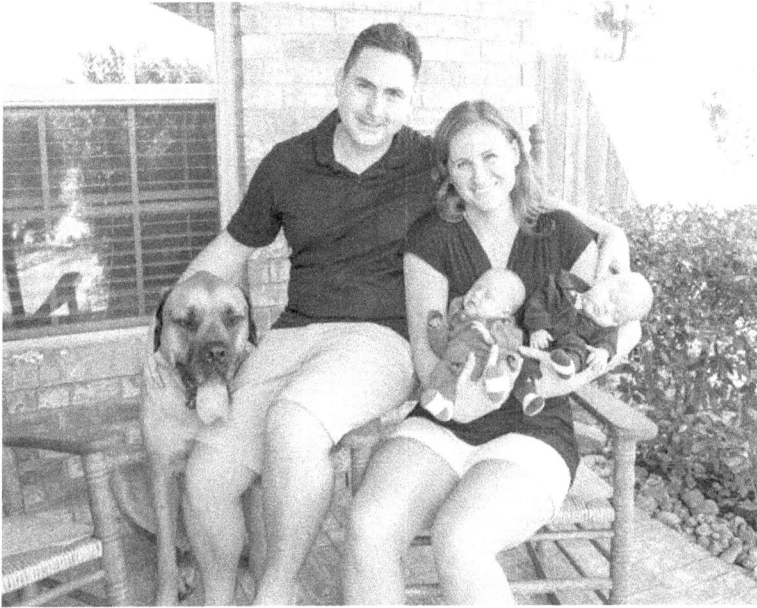

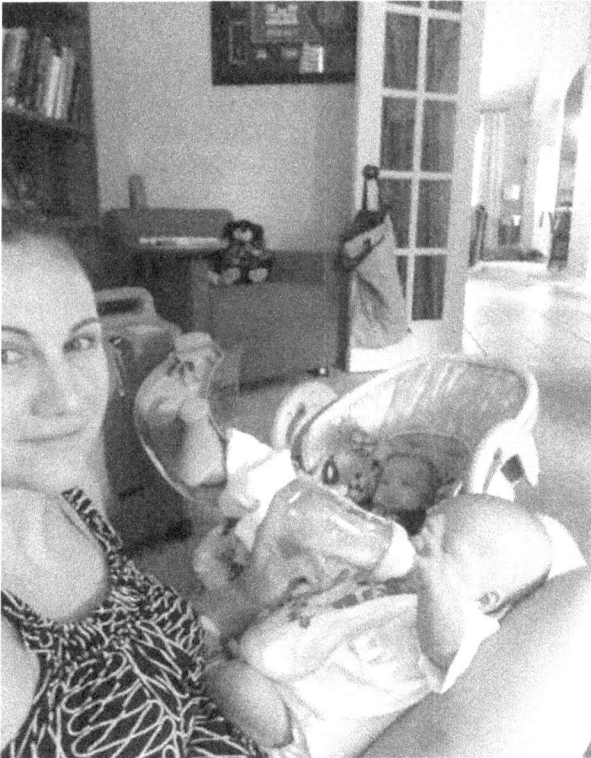

Tiny

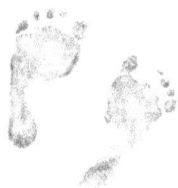

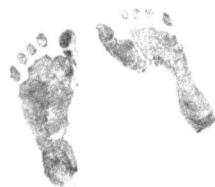

<u>More Emotions</u>

EVEN AFTER THE BOYS CAME HOME FROM the NICU, I was still a roller coaster of emotions. I was happy they were home, and I was worried I would do something to jeopardize their health. Some friends and family desperately wanted us to be able to tell them that everything was fine, the boys were going to be perfect, they were doing everything they were supposed to do, and they were totally out of the woods. While, for the most part, the boys were doing great, we simply could not predict the future and offer that kind of reassurance to our family. Certainly the concerns for their immediate health and our fears and worries had lessened once the boys came home. Now we were less concerned with them simply surviving and more concerned with how much they were eating, how much Chuck was pooping to make sure nothing was going wrong with his gut, and trying to start reaching those milestones that other full term babies had already mastered.

Our worries were much different than those of the parents to a healthy full term baby. I felt as though we had to take advantage of every second they were awake to do tummy time so we could start to close the gap of their adjusted age with them being able to hold their head up and so on. It felt more like every day was filled with physical therapy and not just relaxing cuddle time. I got jealous of photos I saw of new moms lounging with their infants and simply snuggling on the couch because not only was my time now divided between two babies, but all my energy was going into making sure they were catching up to their peers and not "wasting" any time.

* * * * *

Even after the boys were home, some things threw me for a loop that I was not expecting. Before we learned we were pregnant, it felt as though everyone around me was getting pregnant but me. Having fertility problems can be very isolating and sometimes I felt as though I could not turn around without seeing someone pregnant. Some of that feeling certainly went away when I actually got pregnant, but after the boys were born it was difficult to not feel robbed of months of pregnancy I missed out on and feel deprived of healthy babies. After the boys came home, I was not prepared for all the emotions I would feel when friends gave birth to healthy full term babies and even healthy full term twins. I was utterly happy that their babies were healthy and glad they did not have to go through what we had. But I was also jealous. And then guilty for feeling anything but happiness for them. These feelings did not last long, but they were very intense. Recognizing them and validating them helped them pass. It is still hard not to be envious of full term moms-to-be since I will never get to feel what that is like. It is also heart wrenching to hear someone say they want to be induced early or try to start labor early on their own because they are sick of feeling so heavily pregnant. I know what every month, day, and minute that a baby is inside growing can mean to how healthy they are when they are born. I certainly do not know what it is like to be so uncomfortable at 9 months pregnant, but it is still hard to hear moms-to-be wishing their babies could be born earlier than they are ready to be.

* * * * *

Connect with other parents who are going through what you are. In-person support groups and online support groups can be extremely helpful. It was validating to be able to voice my feelings to someone who understood what I was going through and feeling since many parents or family members could not understand my emotions. It is reassuring to feel as though you are not the only one feeling a certain way. I think that helped me move past those emotions. You may not have friends or family who can understand what you are going through or have gone through, but you may find a new friend online who is in an almost identical situation. I now have a friend with twin boys whose medical history is unbelievably similar to my boys' who lives in another state. It is so helpful to talk to her and, although we have yet to met in person, I consider her one of my best friends.

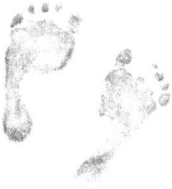

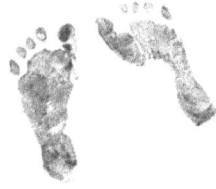

Schedules

WHEN NEWBORNS COME HOME FROM THE hospital, they dictate the schedule. They will either wake to eat or need to be woken to eat, they may play for a short while, and then they sleep again. Somewhere in there you will change their diaper, maybe eat something yourself, possibly try to keep a sibling or two entertained, and if you are absolutely lucky you may get in a nap. I think that is the basic newborn schedule. It is not about what time something happens, more about the flow and the order of things.

We did not have a schedule so much as we had a routine we repeated over and over again throughout the day. We were seeing the pediatrician once a month for a weight check and an RSV shot. It was that second month home during our visit to the pediatrician that he was so pleased with the boys' weights (both around 10 pounds, still gaining over a pound a month). He said we no longer had to wake them every 3 hours as long as they were drinking the same volume in 24 hours that they were currently drinking and that that amount continued to slowly increase. The hope was the boys would sleep a little longer for each stretch but wake hungrier and, therefore, be able to eat the same volume in 24 hours as they currently were eating every 3 hours. Hearing that the boys were doing so well we did not have to wake them as often was exciting, but knowing I was going to be able to (possibly) sleep longer than 2 and a half hours in a row was one of the best things I had ever heard. After 211 days, I was looking forward to spacing my pumping out a bit more and maybe getting a few hours of sleep in a row overnight. I was also extremely nervous that the boys would sleep too much, not be able to drink enough, and their weight would start to drop off.

When we got home I calculated what they would need to drink every 4 hours instead of every 3 and filled their bottles for the next 24 hours to see if they could finish it. This was an easy way to track how they continued to do. After a few days and then weeks, we were able to tweak their schedule to have them drink more during the day and less at night to give them longer stretches of solid sleep overnight. They still needed to be woken, both during the day and at night, but it was starting to resemble more of a schedule and less of a routine.

When the boys first came home, we were most concerned with how much they ate and making sure they got a certain number of bottles of breastmilk and certain number of bottles of formula a day. There was no way I was going to remember what kind of bottle they had already had and what kind was next, especially when they were finally both home, so we needed a chart. Most of the books I had read about twins had recommended using a chart. I was able to combine what I liked best about each chart in the books I had into an excel worksheet and that was what we used. It was nice to have the chart saved on the computer to be able to modify it as things changed. The first iteration had a space next to each hour in the day to record whether the baby got a breastmilk bottle, a formula bottle, or tried breastfeeding, how much they drank, which breast they nursed on, and whether they were wet or dry. Eventually I eliminated the column for nursing and after a few months we were able to eliminate the column for formula. We also added a column for medication when Henry needed it three times a day for reflux and we added a column for baths. We were bathing the boys every other day, but I could never remember if they needed one or not. We kept that chart until their first birthday.

Every few weeks I would print more pages of the chart, one for each day, and we kept the pages in a 3-ring binder where we fed the boys so it was easy to remember to record the information. After their first birthday, we stopped recording everything but Chuck's poops and eye patching. For that I printed a monthly calendar on one sheet of paper and we gave a check mark on that day every time he pooped. I also wrote L or R for which eye was being patched that day since we were alternating the patches.

* * * * *

I have heard some apps are helpful for breastfeeding in general or breastfeeding twins and others for tracking naps, bottles, and whatnot. We had not found one that would allow both parents to enter data independently and then synchronize when the boys came home. At one point my husband was doing the last bottle of the day while I only pumped and immediately went back to bed. For us it was easier for him to record on the paper chart what they had eaten; therefore, when I started again the next day without him, I knew what kind of bottle each baby needed.

* * * * *

Do not listen to anyone who tells you 'never wake a sleeping baby' if you and your pediatrician have a plan that involves waking your baby or babies! I cannot count how many people asked why we could not just let them sleep or told me they did not understand why we were waking them. That was fine with me-they did not need to understand. I understood, as did their pediatrician. Babies reach a certain age and weight when they will naturally wake themselves when they are hungry. How lucky that most babies are born full term and can go home feeding ad lib and wake whenever their little bodies tell them they need to eat. Some premature babies, mine included, did not yet have these cues to wake and eat. Unless they were woken, they would not wake enough during the day to eat enough to keep them growing as much as they needed to. We relied on the guidance of our pediatrician to tell us when we could take away formula and replace it with breastmilk and when the boys could go longer than 3 hours between eating. These were my first micro preemies, but not his, so I trusted him and they continued to grow on his advice.

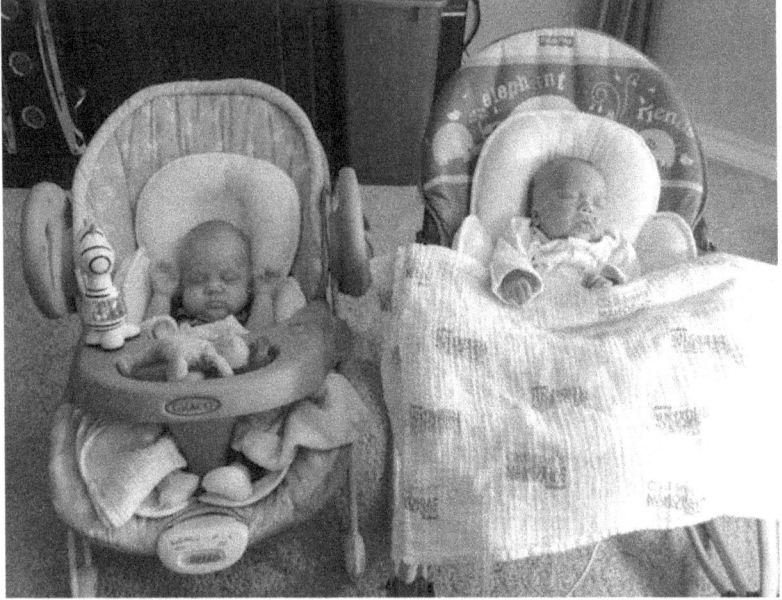

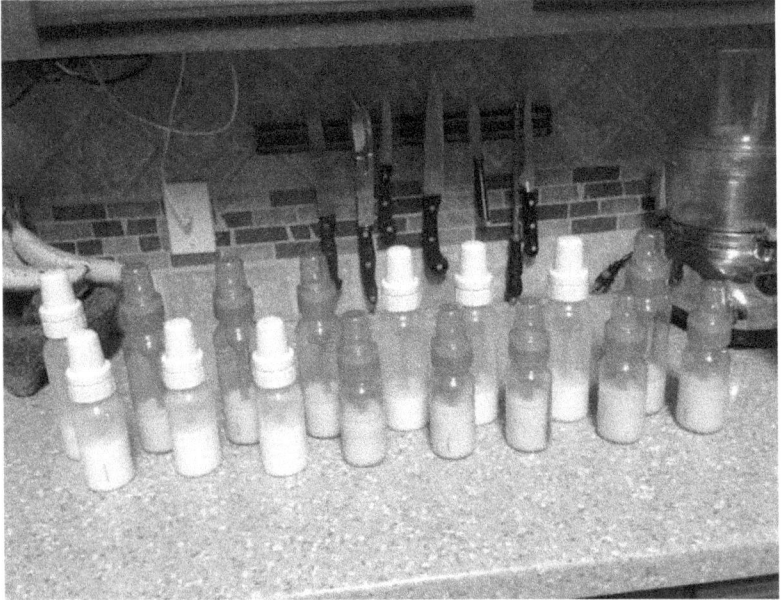

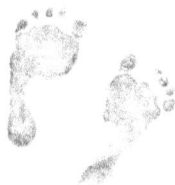

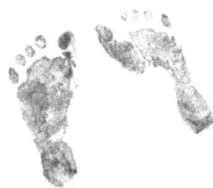

Milestones

IT WAS NOT LONG AFTER THE BOYS CAME HOME that they were actually beginning to accomplish the same milestones as "regular" babies. The boys were smiling, starting to support some of their weight on their legs when we held them, and starting to sit up in the Bumbo® chair or in Boppy® pillow. They even grew out of newborn clothes and out of newborn diapers. Some of these are milestones babies master in the hospital or very soon after, but even at 5 months or older we felt as though they were each hard won for us and very important. The calendars I had started as soon as the babies were born had recorded things from the NICU such as "off the vent," "first surgery," "first sponge bath," "first time held," "PICC line out," "first time in clothes," and all their various CPAP and cannula tries and those sorts of things. I was now starting to be able to use the stickers that came with the calendars to mark their accomplishments of standing assisted, sitting assisted, smiles and those sorts of things.

One big milestone was moving some parts of the day from our room to their own room. Since they were now awake for longer and longer after each bottle and starting to really enjoy tummy time, we decided that rather than bringing all the baby toys downstairs to the office where we had been feeding the boys we would move playtime (and therefore feeding time also) upstairs in their room. They were also finally big enough for the cloth diapers we had planned to use and Chuck was now healed enough that I felt comfortable using them with him. His surgeon had said that disposable diapers wick moisture better due to the chemicals they contain and his incision would initially heal better with disposable diapers. He was now healed enough that we could try the cloth on him. It had been easy to keep disposable diapers and wipes downstairs, but the cloth diapers would involve more so it made sense to move the diaper changing to their real changing table where everything was ready and had been waiting for them. After about a month and a half of sleeping nights in the mini crib in our room, we started putting them to sleep during the night upstairs in their room. They were still napping during the day on the couch on their tummies at this point since Chuck was still on oxygen, but most of our day was now spent in their room having a bottle, pumping, and playing before they needed a nap and I brought them downstairs again.

* * * * *

Do not forget to mark milestones on a calendar (or somehow) so that you can not only record them to look back on later but also for your pediatrician, if necessary. Our pediatrician asked us to use a common monthly milestone chart and to record the month our boys did things to make sure that even if they were behind on accomplishing things, they were making their own steady progress. I made a copy and brought him the chart every month when we went for our visit.

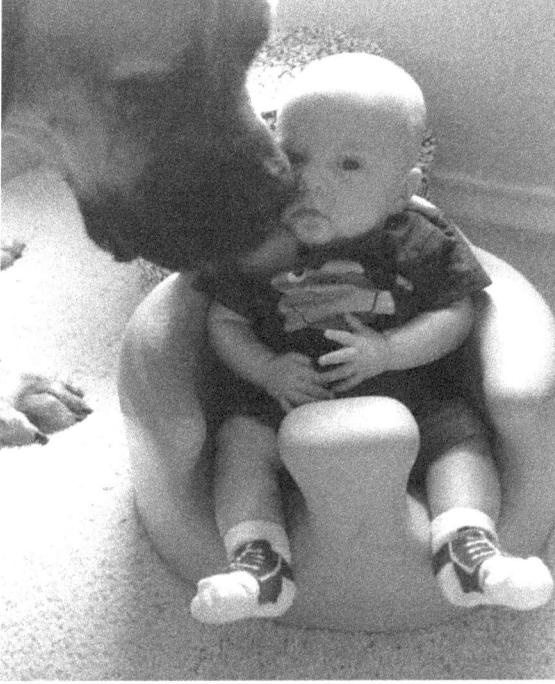

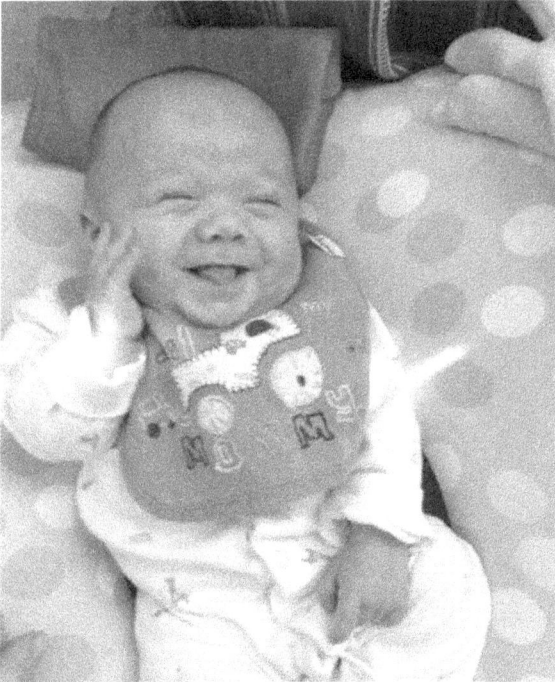

Tiny

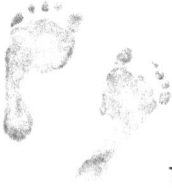

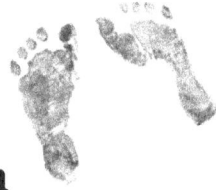

Early Intervention

EARLY INTERVENTION IS A NATIONALLY AND STATE funded program that varies in name from state to state. Our NICU nurses, neonatologists and social worker told us to call our state program, Early Childhood Intervention (ECI, run in our area by Easter Seals®), as soon as the boys were home so that they could be evaluated and possibly receive services such as physical or occupational therapy. Qualification standards also vary from state to state. In some states a baby qualifies for EI based on birth weight alone. In our state, babies as young as ours were evaluated based on their actual birthday and their adjusted age. They either needed to show a lag in development compared with their adjusted age or have been diagnosed with one of a long list of prequalifying diagnosis in order to qualify for ECI.

The evaluators came to our house a month after both boys came home. At that point they were 6 months old but only 2 months adjusted. Since there is not too much a 2 month old should be doing, they did not show a significant lag behind that age. They were essentially expected at that point to be doing things a baby who had recently been born should be doing, and they were doing those things. Henry did not have any diagnoses that automatically qualified him for services, but Chuck had a "failure to thrive" diagnosis on his discharge paperwork for the period of time that he was not gaining weight awaiting surgery. The fact that he was now thriving did not matter because he could qualify based on that diagnosis. Henry was not going to receive services, but Chuck qualified for 4 visits per month from a services coordinator at a cost to us adjusted based on our income. Our insurance covered the cost of the evaluation and then we paid a low cost monthly for the visits.

Even though only Chuck qualified, it was fairly impossible to separate the boys so they both benefited from the visits. When our coordinator visited, I was able to use all the information she gave me concerning things that I could be doing to help Chuck with his milestones and use them with Henry as well. From the milestone list I was keeping for the pediatrician, I had a good idea of what they should be accomplishing but I did not know how to help them. Our coordinator gave me tricks and tips for tummy time and for grasping toys. She also suggested bottle holders to help the boys hold their own bottle and (for the most part) feed themselves by 9 months old. That suggestion alone was worth its weight in gold, because I could finally pump, burp and attend to them while they ate but not have to also hold two bottles for their entire feed. She suggested some toys that helped reach certain milestones and gave me strategies to help them roll, crawl and walk.

ECI was certainly a resource of which we took full advantage. It was also nice to have another set of eyes on the boys, someone who sees lots of babies, to let me know what was normal and what was not. At one point we both noticed Chuck favoring his left foot and left hand and she scheduled an evaluation from a physical therapist. The physical therapist said how impressed she was with how the boys were doing. When she heard she was going to evaluate a 24 weeker, she had prepared for the need for a wheelchair or braces and things like that, but when she arrived and saw him walking against the wall she was thrilled. She explained that when Chuck came home and his oxygen saturation was better on his right side and so we laid him on his right side to sleep, he had more visual access to his left hand and foot and therefore he developed a preference for them. She was able to give us some strategies for working both sides of Chuck's body so he did not favor his left hand or foot. He did not qualify for additional services or any kind of ongoing physical therapy, which was great.

Since the boys continued to slowly make up the disparity between what they could do and what their full term peers were doing, Chuck had his annual review and was caught up enough to not qualify for the program anymore. That was great news because it meant that we were on track to continue to catch up, hopefully by their second birthday. It also made me a little nervous that someone would not be checking in with us to make sure I was not missing anything. But an EI evaluation can be done at any time, so if ever in the future (up to age 3) we feel as though there is a need we can call ECI again and someone could come reevaluate either of the boys.

* * * * *

Sometimes scheduling the initial Early Intervention evaluation can take a few weeks. Call early (even before your baby is out of the hospital) and call back if your phone calls are not being returned. Many children are in EI programs, and persistence pays off.

* * * * *

The sliding payment scale, in our state, changed during the year we received services. Luckily we were grandfathered in so our payments did not change during the 12 months we received services, but after the yearly evaluation, if we had continued to receive services, our monthly payment would have increased 700%. If we require services in the future we will certainly consider ECI, but we will also look into private therapy because it might be covered fully or partially by insurance and might be less expensive.

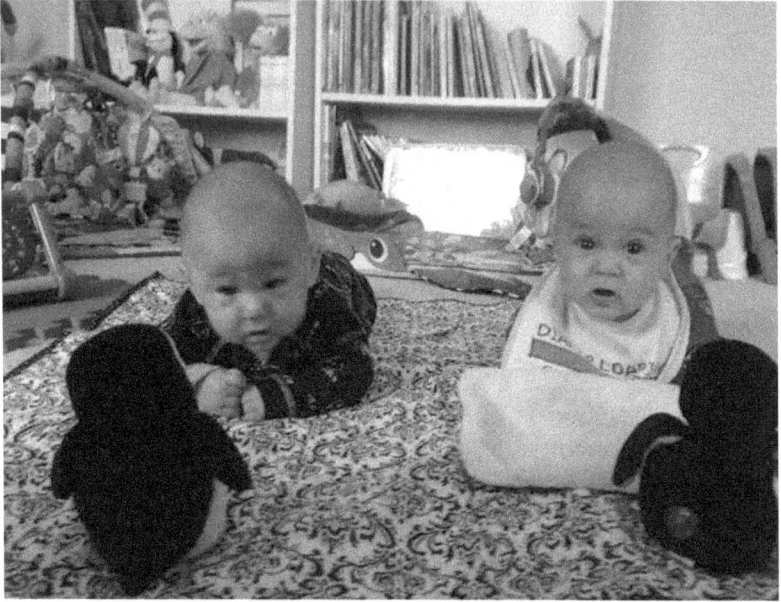

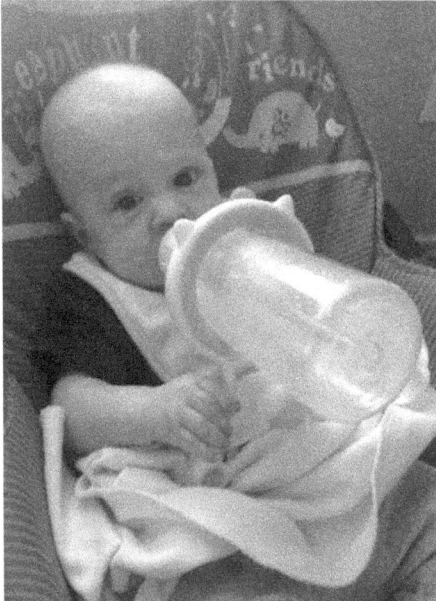

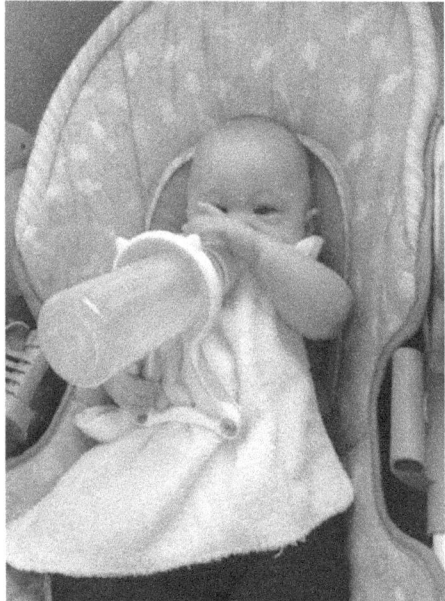

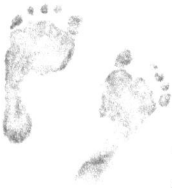

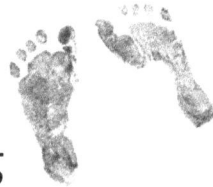

<u>Lots of Growing</u>

THE FIRST MONTHS THAT THE BOYS WERE home were filled with lots of firsts and lots of growing. We invited the boys' primary nurses for lunch at our house since they had not seen the boys in over 3 months. It was fun to show them how much the boys had grown. It was nice to visit with other adults too, especially for me since I was not leaving the house during the day. I would go to the grocery store when the boys were sleeping on a weekend, which was about the only getting out of the house I was doing. We were not going on walks yet because Chuck's oxygen made it tough, and they were only awake for such a short period of time that I tried to get in as much tummy time as possible. Therefore, visiting with the nurses was very enjoyable.

The boys were finally starting to have nights where they would sleep for 4 hours in a row, wake for a bottle, and sleep another 4 hours. That was a huge milestone. I was now only pumping when they were eating, and we were down to about 6 bottles/pumps a day. We also had to buy larger bottles that held more since they were eating almost 30 ounces a day. They both decided to laugh for the first time a few days apart, which was really fun. Also, Chuck had a visit to the pediatrician for a weigh in and was doing so well he got to ditch his last formula bottle and was on only breastmilk. Throughout the fall my pumping was able to keep up with what they were eating in 24 hours, but my supply was not increasing as it (ideally) would have been had they been breastfeeding. I tried many things to assist with increasing my supply but did not succeed. Eventually they surpassed what I could produce in a day and I started dipping into our frozen stash.

By the end of the fall Chuck no longer required oxygen during his bottles at all and was doing so well on such little oxygen during his sleep that we put him back on the monitor and off the oxygen during the night to see if he could do it on his own. I slept on the floor of the boys' room for a week to be close enough to silence the monitor quickly if it went off and make sure he recovered right away if his oxygen dipped down. He did great, and around Thanksgiving he did not need to go back on the oxygen for any reason. We had a follow up appointment with his doctor monitoring the oxygen a few weeks later, and they felt confident with how he was doing that they wrote the order to have the oxygen removed.

Although both boys were doing great on breastmilk, Henry started to have some reflux issues that were not resolving themselves. The amount of spit up and the frequency that he was spitting up did not matter if he was still gaining weight. However, he started to spit up and then be in so much pain that he did not want to finish his bottle. At his checkup a few days later, he had not gained as much weight as we would have liked. Therefore he went on medication for reflux and after about a week we noticed it making a difference. He was still spitting up frequently and a fairly good volume, but he was returning to the bottle to finish, which meant he was getting more calories than the month before. As he gained weight we had to go up on the medication dosage once, but other than that he did well with it and the prescription made a huge difference for the few months that he needed it. Before his first birthday we were able to wean him off without the discomfort returning, and he was able to stay off for good and continue to gain about a pound a month, as Chuck was.

* * * * *

SSpitting up can be completely normal, and even a lot of spit up is not worrisome as long as baby is continuing to gain weight. However, reflux that causes pain is very common in preemies and can hinder their desire to finish a bottle and therefore gain weight. Some doctors recommend rice cereal by mouth or bottle to help the liquid stay in the tummy and others recommend medication. I had hoped to avoid medication, but it made a huge difference and Henry did not need to be on it for very long. Make sure you talk to the doctor before experimenting with rice cereal, as it is not recommended for babies until a certain age as to not hurt the fragile digestive system.

* * * * *

We had purchased hard foam mats to cover the carpeting in the boys' room, where we were feeding them, and it helped protect the carpet from all Henry's spitting up. We later moved the mats to the play room, and they still help with straw cup spills and goldfish cracker crumbs.

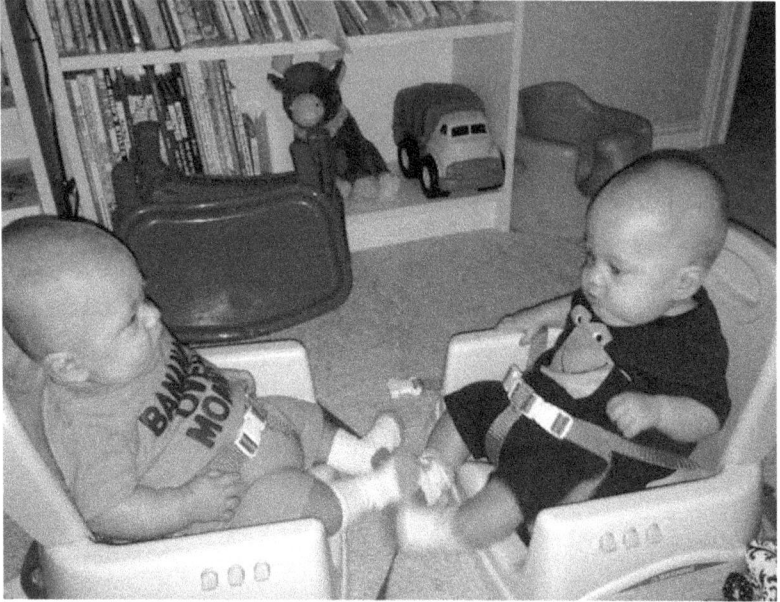

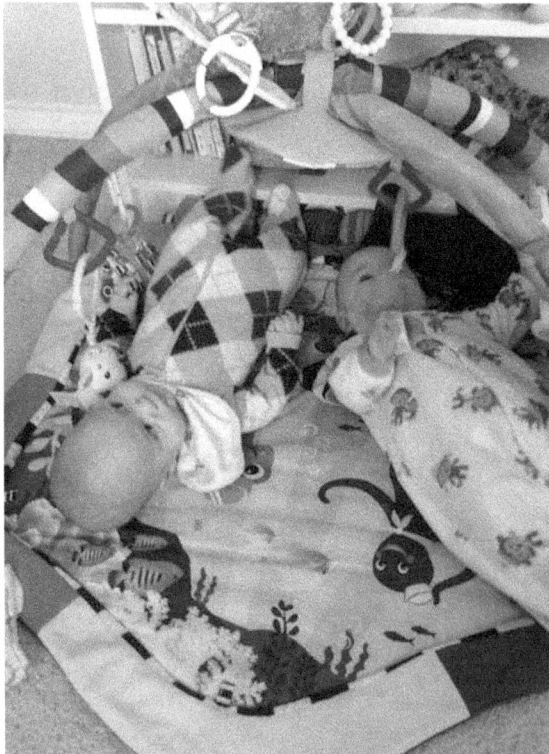

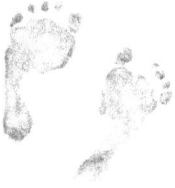

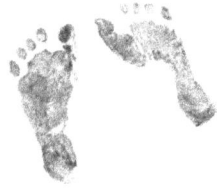

First Babysitter and Weekend with Dad

BY THE MIDDLE OF THE WINTER THE BOYS were starting to roll a bit and playtime began to last longer and become more interactive. They continued to be weighed every month when they got their RSV shot and kept up their pound a month gain. They still were not on the regular baby height/weight curves, but they were making progress on their own curve and headed towards catching up, which was okay. They were doing so well I was able to take a weekend away and fly to the opposite coast for a family wedding. Everyone was disappointed the boys could not join me, but they understood that traveling in the height of flu season during one of the busiest airport times of the year was too big of a chance for them to get sick. We needed a babysitter to allow me to leave for the airport a few hours before my husband got home from work, and we lucked out that one of our primary nurses was available. It made leaving them for the first time with someone else as easy as it could have been. Not only was it someone who was already familiar with them, but she was probably even more qualified to take care of them than I was. It allowed me to leave without worrying. I was still pumping, but I had enough of a stash in the freezer that I did not want the hustle of trying to bring the milk home. I was able to borrow my neighbor's travel pump so that I could both plug it in when I was at the hotel and also use the batteries at the airport.

I was able to upgrade to first class for a very small fee for the flight to the wedding. That was a relief for me because it ensured there was room in the overhead bins for my dress and also meant I would inconvenience fewer people when I needed to use plane bathroom to pump. I told the flight attendant I would be pumping for about 20 minutes before I went into the bathroom; therefore, she was not concerned and could let anyone that was waiting know that I would be awhile. Apparently I should have let my seat mate know also, because when I came back he was very concerned and asked if I was alright. I said I was still breastfeeding and I had to pump. He laughed and very nicely said he did not mean to pry, but he was a doctor and always kept an eye out for anyone looking queasy in case he was needed. He said he had not thought I looked ill so he could not imagine what had gone on in the bathroom for so long. He asked how old my child was and was surprised to hear I had twins and how early they had been born. As it turned out, more than 20 years before, he had been part of the trials for one of the medications for lung development that the boys had received when they were first born. He said the study was actually stopped and all the babies were given the drug instead of half being given the placebo because the doctors saw what a difference the drug was making and ethically could not withhold it from the other sick babies. It was incredible to hear and such a coincidence to be sitting next to him.

Since I was flying in the night before the wedding, there was not much time to do anything after landing but get to the hotel, pump, go to bed, and wake up for a full day of wedding prep and wedding. Since the wedding was being held at the hotel where we were staying, sneaking away to pump was as easy as it could have been. The only hiccup was that I could not zip up my strapless maid of honor dress myself and therefore during the reception I had to call my mom on my cell phone to come help me when I was done pumping. Other than that, it was fairly easy to pump and dump and clean the pumping supplies every 4 hours.

The ceremony was beautiful and flawless. The reception had just begun and I was about to stand to make my toast when my husband texted me that Henry had a fever and wanted to double check what to do. Since the boys had been so fragile when they came home, we had been advised that any fever over 104 was something we should immediately go to the emergency room for and anything less was something we should call the doctor for to get the proper dosage of Tylenol®. Luckily Henry's fever was not so high he needed to go to the emergency room; therefore, I told my husband to call the doctor's number and wait for the on call pediatrician to let him know about the medication. I texted him back just in the nick of time to stand and give my toast. I then handed the microphone to the best man for his toast and discreetly picked my phone back up and walked out of the reception room and down the hall to call my husband and get a few more details about how Henry was feeling. I was not a nervous wreck, but I was concerned that neither of the boys had had a fever since they had been discharged and if either one of them had contracted RSV it would likely mean a hospital stay and a very sick baby. I was worried and hoped to hear that Henry had gone back to sleep easily. I needed a few minutes to gather myself and a bit of reassurance from my husband. What I did not need was to be told to calm down and put my phone away when I returned to the table. It is difficult for others to realize how serious something may actually be if they have only had full term healthy children. What for some kids may be very run of the mill for others can mean a trip to the hospital and a life-threatening sickness. Unfortunately the bride overheard that Henry was sick and was, of course, concerned. I tried to reassure everyone, including myself, that he would be fine, but that I was anxious to hear that the doctor agreed that Tylenol® was all he needed.

* * * * *

Your baby will eventually get sick with some bug or another after discharge. You probably will be extremely anxious and scared. Most likely everything will turn out fine, but it is normal to immediately fear the worst. Your pediatrician will understand and will not begrudge you when you make appointments for simple fevers and sniffles that a fourth time parent of a full term baby would never feel the need to go to the pediatrician with. That is okay. Guess what? Your baby is different and you are allowed to be scared. The second or third fever or cough or cold will be less and less scary. But the first one will be pretty terrifying.

* * * * *

Do not tell the parent of a preemie or micro preemie to calm down or not freak out or that your baby had fevers all the time and you know they are not a big deal, because for preemies and micro preemies they are a big deal. It is a big deal for the parent and it is a big deal for the baby. Instead, validate their feelings and try to help them think positively. Simply acknowledging that they are scared and you hope the baby is well soon goes a long way.

* * * * *

Emergency rooms, sick day visits to the pediatrician, and on call after hours doctors and nurses are there for a reason. Use them. Certainly, you do not have to call for every runny nose, but if you think something is wrong then you should call. It is much better to be reassured something is normal or can be treated with over the counter medication than to be up worried sick all night watching over a sleeping baby. You may be up worried anyway, but it helps to get that second opinion that things will be okay and that you are doing the right thing.

* * * * *

Be sure to write down the Tylenol® doses your doctor advises before administering medication, as it can be hard to remember what you are told for the next dose.

LUCKILY HENRY FELT FINE IN THE MORNING and only needed some medication to bring down his fever and some extra cuddling. He did not end up catching RSV and he did not need to go to the hospital. I was very relieved to come home the next day and be with both of them. Chuck ended up catching his virus and got a fever a few days later. We, therefore, doled out the Tylenol® and spent New Year's Eve going to sleep well before the ball dropped, waking up for bottles and pumping, and going back to sleep. It was nice to have 2013 behind us and look forward to 2014.

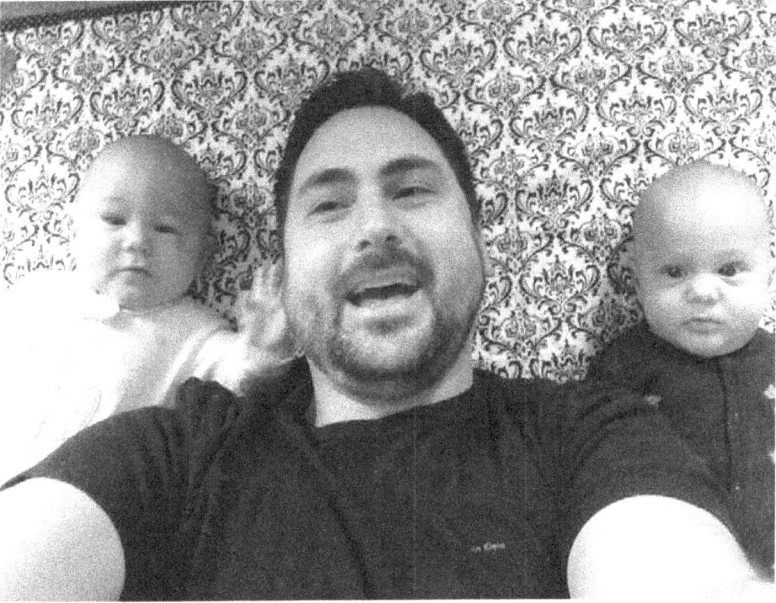

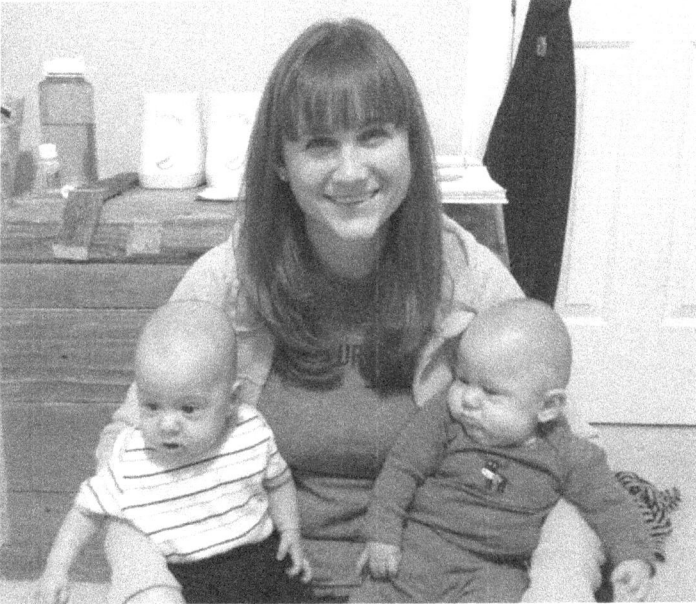

Tiny

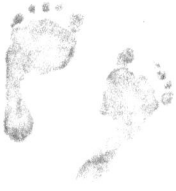

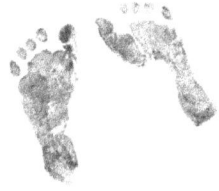

Naps and Sleeping

THE BIGGEST CHANGE OF THE NEW YEAR WAS the boys' sleeping arrangement. The boys had napped downstairs on the couch during the day because they slept better on their stomachs and I could watch them during nap time that way. However, they both started to wake up an hour into their nap, which should have been much longer to keep them happy, and nothing was able to get them back to sleep. After some internet research and sleep book reading, I decided they were waking up after one sleep cycle and were not able to soothe themselves back to sleep. After a week of horrible naps, trying to get them back to sleep in the swing, and begging them to sleep longer in general, I gave up and overhauled their sleeping arrangement.

Most any baby book or sleep book will tell you that naps should be just like overnight sleep-in the same place, in the same way and starting from day 1. That was not possible for us since Chuck's oxygen had dictated their sleeping location and position until this point. I figured it was worth a try to pretend they were newborns and give them a fresh start sleeping how we would have preferred them to sleep when they came home from the hospital. Ideally they would have napped on their backs in their crib, the same way they were sleeping overnight. I decided we would try making all their naps in their crib. They would each be in their own crib since they were now starting to kick and move and wake each other up during overnight sleep. Also, we would let them try to soothe themselves since they were now old enough and capable of putting their pacifier back in their mouth or using a fist or thumb to soothe themselves back to sleep.

The first night in separate cribs went fine and they did not seem to notice anything was different. Although I was still feeding at least one bottle during the night, they would wake to be changed, drink it and go right back to sleep. They were sleeping 12 hours total, so we could not complain there. Henry took to sleeping naps on his back in his crib like a champ, but Chuck was still waking up half way through a nap, would wake Henry up, and then it became a two screaming baby nightmare. I took Chuck out of his crib for naps and put him in the pack and play in our laundry room because it was dark, the vent made great white noise, and it was air conditioned and cool. That way he could have a chance to soothe himself back to sleep if he needed to and would not wake Henry. It worked amazingly well, and they were both back to the long naps they needed to keep them happy.

* * * * *

Do whatever works for naps and overnight sleep in the beginning; sleep habits can always be corrected later. Sure, it would be ideal to bring babies home and have them go to sleep on their backs in a crib for every nap and all their night sleep and never need a pacifier and never cry it out and just be a dream. I have never heard of a baby doing that, especially not a preemie or a micro preemie. Lots of preemies have reflux and need to be kept upright for a half hour or so after they eat. One person trying to keep two tiny babies upright for a half hour after they eat when all they want to do as newborns is immediately go back to sleep can be impossible. Use all the tools at your disposal and do not feel badly about using them. Swings, bouncy seats, and MamaRoo®s can all keep babies at a good angle for reflux and allow them to sleep. Nothing made me happier than when one of the other moms in my multiples group told me her son slept in a swing for naps until he was 7 months old. I suddenly did not feel guilty about letting Henry nap in a swing when it was the only thing that made him happy. Even though we let him nap on his tummy while I was watching him or in a swing, the transition to sleeping on his back in his crib for naps and overnight sleep went as smoothly as could be. I thought "giving in" and letting them nap or sleep on their tummies or in a swing would ruin their sleep and make for horrific screaming and crying when we eventually needed them to sleep in their cribs, but the crying never came and they did great.

EVEN THOUGH THEY WERE MUCH OLDER THAN some babies who slept through the night, our boys still needed a bottle or two overnight because they were still trying to catch up in weight and growing so fast that they needed all the calories they could get. They were rock stars about waking for a bottle and immediately going back to sleep during the overnight hours. They never confused night for day and never thought it was playtime when it was middle of the night bottle time, which was great. I kept the lights as low as possible (sometimes only using a light from downstairs, which gave me just enough light to change them and feed them) to help them stay sleepy, drink, and pass out again.

* * * * *

During overnight feeds, I tried to keep the lights as low as possible. At first, I replaced the changing table light in their room with the lowest wattage I could find, but even that was pretty bright. After a few months I realized I could change them and give them a bottle using only my phone light and the microwave light from downstairs. I think the minimal amount of light helped them to never think it was playtime and to always go right back to sleep.

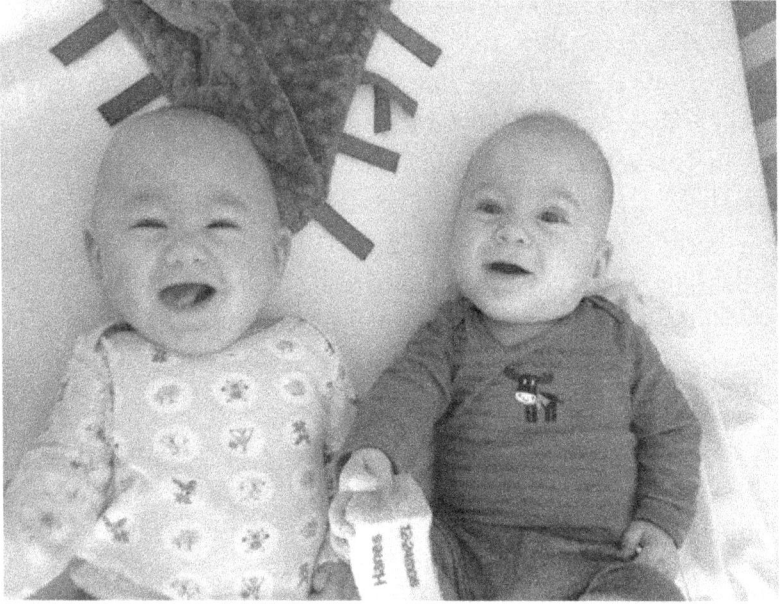

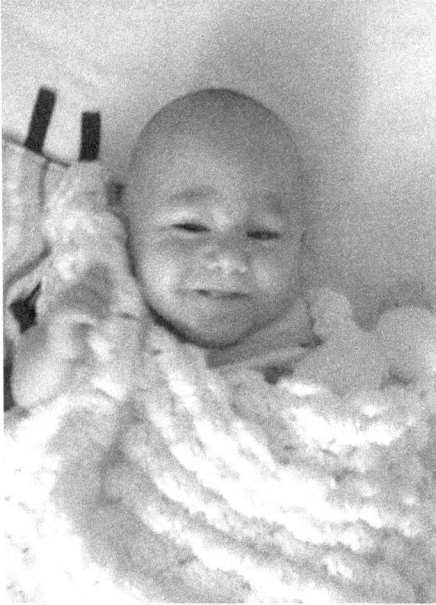

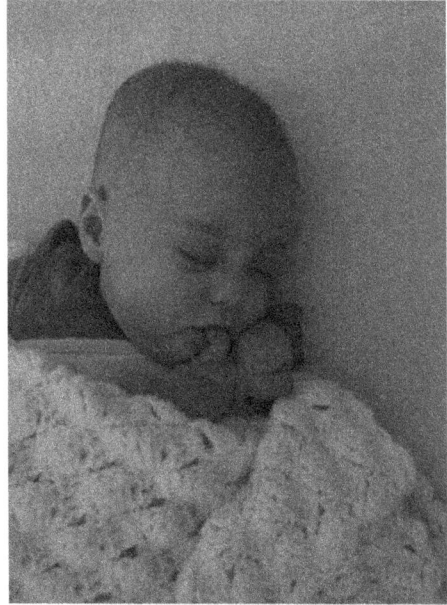

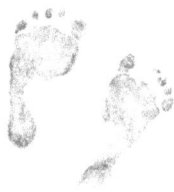

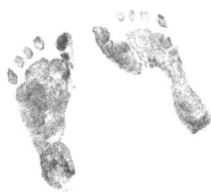

Solid Food

THE NEW YEAR ALSO BROUGHT NEW FOOD. I had planned on waiting until the boys were 6 months old, as recommended by the American Association of Pediatrics, to start solid food because starting earlier can sometimes negatively affect the baby's sensitive digestive tract. We were already very conscious of Chuck and digestion because of his surgeries. Also, contrary to popular belief, starting food months early has been studied and shown not to make a difference in helping babies sleep through the night. We were not interested in the boys sleeping any longer anyway since they still needed to wake for a bottle to help them continue to grow on track. We waited until the boys were more than 5 months old adjusted (they were actually almost 9 months old in reality), and the pediatrician encouraged us to start solids to help weigh the milk down and hopefully help Henry's reflux.

I looked up recommended first foods and decided to start with avocado, pumpkin, apple sauce, and oatmeal rather than the traditional rice cereal. I thought foods naturally rich in iron and zinc would be helpful since the boys were on a multivitamin from being deficient in those while in the hospital. I knew they would be on a multivitamin until they were off breastmilk since breastmilk is naturally low in iron, but I hoped more iron in their diet could help them. Chuck loved his first bite of avocado, but Henry made a very troublesome face. After a few days of trying food after their morning bottle, Henry came around and did better than Chuck. ECI reminded me that "food before one is just for fun," and we did not want to push Chuck too hard if he was not ready. Breastmilk was providing all the calories and nutrients that the boys needed to grow and develop, and we did not want to force solids on Chuck before he was ready as to not create an aversion.

We started out offering solid food after their bottle; therefore, they received all the important calories and nutrition from the breast-milk.. We started offering puree once a day. We did three days on each food to make sure neither of the boys had a reaction to it and then went on to the next food. Eventually we fed them twice a day up until their first birthday. I am glad that there was not a lot of pressure to make sure they were getting a certain amount of real food and that I knew they were getting all their required nutrition just from their bottles because at first it was very difficult to fit that solid food feeding in every day. Some days it would feel like I blinked, and the end of the day was upon us and I had forgotten to give them anything solid.

Since we were doing almost everything for the boys upstairs, we fed them upstairs initially too. We tried the Bumbo® chairs first because I thought since they were eating they should be in a chair. We tried their high chairs after that. That was a big mistake. The kind of high chairs we got were "space savers" so they attached to a regular chair and were more of a booster with a tray than an actual reclined and padded high chair. We put them on the floor upstairs when we tried them. They required a lot more strength and balance to sit up in them than the Bumbo®s or the reclining bouncy chairs the boys had their bottles in. It was obvious the boys could not sit up and eat at the same time when we tried them. I am grateful I had a random conversation with one of the moms in my MoMs group who did a lot of occupational therapy and had great advice about feeding babies. She said if they were doing fine in the Bumbo®s or even in the vibrating chairs where they had their bottles, there was no reason they could not eat solid food in those. As soon as I talked to her I felt much better, put the high chairs away for later, and went back to the vibrating chairs for solids. They supported the boys and enabled them to relax and concentrate on eating. Chuck was still not as ready as Henry for solid food all the time and some days he only had a bite or two. We made sure not to force it because lots of gagging can cause an aversion. Slowly he got better and better and more receptive to solid food and by their first birthday they were eating solids twice a day every day.

* * * * *

Do not be afraid to try again or skip days when first starting solid food. This is not something to get stressed out about.

AT THEIR 12 MONTH CHECKUP, THE PEDIATRICIAN said it was the time to use food as the main source of nutrition and begin three meals a day of nutritious food and give milk afterwards. We still kept the boys on formula (transition formula) until they were 12 months adjusted (15 months old). We introduced milk, both cow and goat, but we settled on goat because I was able to find that Trader Joe's® humanely raised goat milk was actually higher in calories and fat than organic cow's milk at my grocery store. Since milk is traditionally recommended for toddlers because of its vitamin D, calories and fat, I thought this was the best choice for us. The boys were on a vitamin that already had vitamin D and folic acid so I was not worried about them missing anything cow's milk provided. I was anxious to ditch the milk as soon as possible in favor of real foods and water, even if as soon as possible was going to be age two, and, therefore, I gave the lower end of the recommended number of ounces a day. At the boys' 12 month checkup they were doing great so I lowered the number of ounces a day, and still at their 15 month checkup they were right on track and had gained a pound and a half each in 3 months so we lowered the amount again.

* * * * *

For preemies or micro preemies calories are very important. I was glad I asked our pediatrician and was instructed at first to always give solid food after a bottle to make sure the boys were filling up on high calorie breastmilk and solid food was like dessert.

* * * * *

I made big batches of baby food and froze them so all we had to do was pull it out of the freezer every few days. I used my regular food processor and had no problems. I have heard good things about baby food making systems, but I felt we did not need one. I loved the silicone ice cube trays for initially freezing and then popped the frozen cubes out like ice cubes and stored them in zip top bags in our deep freezer.

* * * * *

Later, when the boys were off bottles and eating solid food full time we did a lot of things to ensure every calorie was a good calorie. They ate cooked eggs with cream cheese and veggies (like a quiche), they had a smoothie I made twice a day with goat milk, peanut butter, bananas, and coconut oil, and they ate grilled cheese with butter and steamed veggies drizzled with olive oil. I think this helped a lot in maintaining the one pound a month gain all the way until they were about 15 months old.

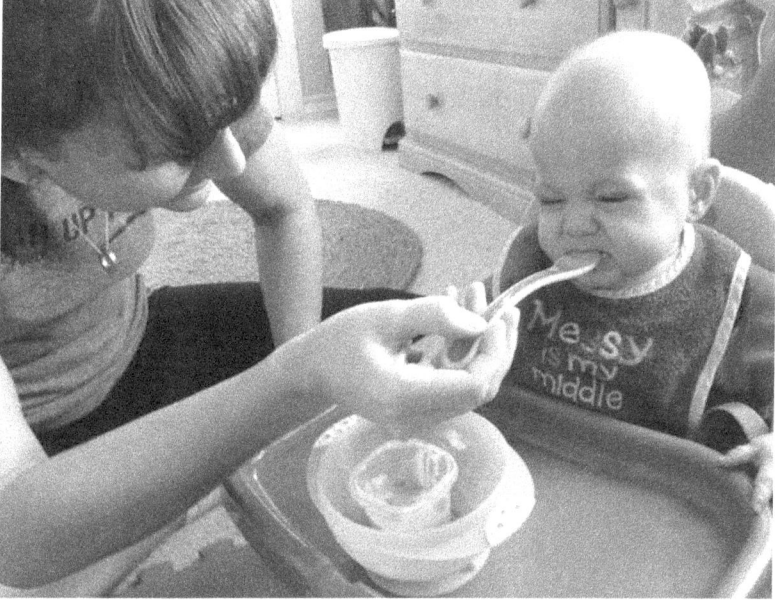

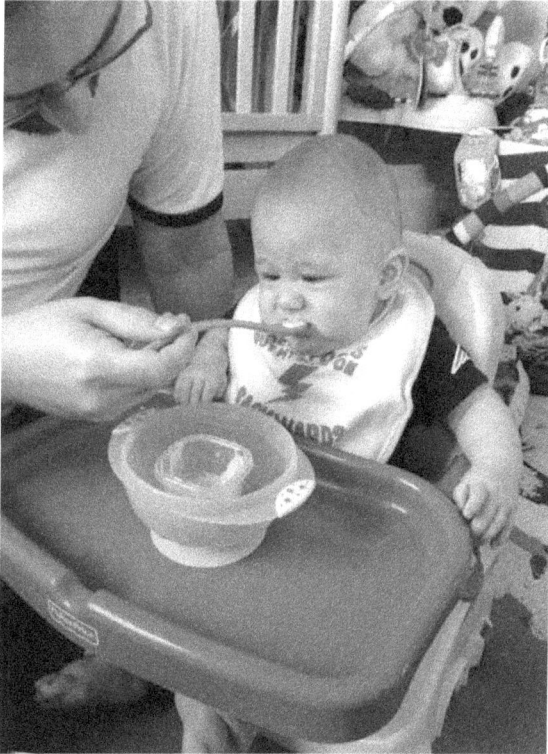

Tiny

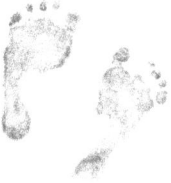

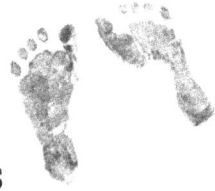

Meeting Milestones

THE BOYS WERE CONTINUING TO CATCH UP with their milestones. We were lucky in that they continued to measure somewhere between their actual age and their adjusted age in terms of when they would hit the common milestones, each month inching closer to their actual age. Chuck began to Army crawl over the winter, a full month before Henry did, and he was constantly working at getting places and using his knees and arms. Henry, on the other hand, never attempted to crawl until one day he decided to get up on his hands and knees and do it perfectly. This proved to be fairly common with the boys and milestones. Chuck did many things before Henry and then had to work to perfect them, while Henry waited longer but did them more confidently the first time.

* * * * *

It is hard not to compare your twins or your baby to someone else's baby who is the same age. Baby books will tell you that every baby grows at their own pace and that comparing is never a good idea. A lot of time during their first year we felt as though our boys were behind our friends' babies who were the same age. It was also tough not to compare the boys to each other and wonder why one was doing something the other was not. Sure enough, they each mastered things at their own pace and continued to catch up to their peers.

* * * * *

It was great when friends and family supported us by making a big deal out of the boys meeting milestones at their own pace and never asking "can they do this yet?" or comparing them to other kids.

* * * * *

Do not feel disappointed at well baby checkups when the nurse asks you questions about what your baby is doing. The questions are based on actual age and not adjusted age. For the first few well baby check-ups, the questions we were asked were a joke and the boys were not doing anything she asked. It might have been discouraging if the doctor then had not come in to tell us how great the boys were progressing and how pleased he was with what they had accomplished. Make sure you do not let someone who does not know the entire situation make you feel as though your baby should be doing more than they are.

ONE THING WE BROUGHT TO OUR PEDIATRICIAN'S attention during a monthly visit was Chuck's eyes turning in to the center intermittently. "Lazy eye" or Strabismus is fairly common with preemies and full term babies. Henry had one eye that turned in for about a month and then it self-corrected. Chuck's affected both eyes and was obvious enough that we went ahead and made the appointment with his ophthalmologist two months earlier than she had asked us to so he could be seen for it. I have family history of this on both sides, and it was more hereditary than something having to do with being premature. Henry needed to be seen also and the ophthalmologist was pleased enough with him that he graduated to seeing a regular pediatric optometrist at three years old. She was able to tell that Chuck had both Strabismus and Amblyopia because his eyes would sometimes turn inward and they focused in two slightly different places. He essentially chose one to look through and the other turned in. This caused him to have a significant reduction in the amount of, if any, depth perception he had. Chuck got a prescription for glasses with a different prescription in each lens to allow his eyes to focus together. The hope was that glasses, along with putting a patch over one eye every day for a few hours, would correct the problem. He would always have to wear glasses (or contact lenses, or get LASIK when he was much older), but it would help strengthen each eye individually and hopefully eliminate the lazy eye.

Chuck began wearing glasses before his first birthday. We got a lot of comments from strangers asking if they were real glasses or just for fun. I do not know who would torture their infant by forcing them to wear glasses unnecessarily. We spent a lot of time explaining that they were indeed real glasses and he needed them to see. The patching helped to a degree, but not enough for him to avoid surgery to correct it permanently. He will continue to wear glasses and we will continue to patch to try to allow him to have the most depth perception that he can possible have.

* * * * *

The ophthalmologist may need to dilate your baby's eyes in the NICU or during a visit. This can take a few rounds of eye drops that are a few minutes apart and then up to a 40 minute wait for the drops to take effect. The second time we went to the doctor I had a plan to entertain my boys during this time. Make sure you either take a walk, or feed, or have toys.

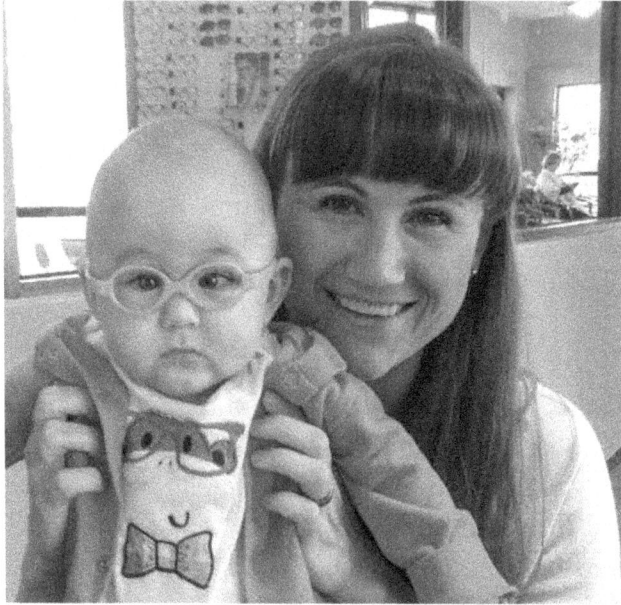

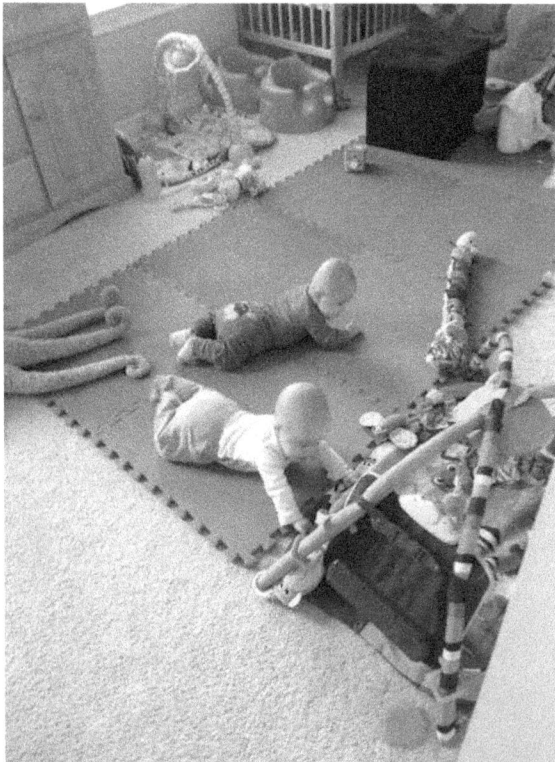

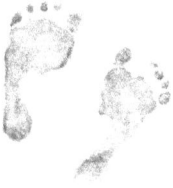

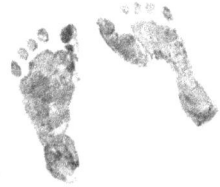

Back to the Hospital

WE WERE VERY LUCKY THAT WE MADE IT almost entirely through flu season only having to bring Henry to the pediatrician for one sick visit when he had ear infections in both ears. Then a month before their first birthday Chuck caught a stomach bug. He started throwing up a few times in the morning, and seemed to feel crummy. I took both boys to the pediatrician by myself for the first time to make sure it was not serious. The pediatrician said he looked good, that it probably was just a virus, and that the major concern would be dehydration. He advised us to buy some Pedialyte® to give him if he threw up his milk. He told me to monitor his diapers to make sure they were nice and wet but thought he would start to feel better that day.

All day Chuck seemed to be doing better, and we told the pediatrician so when he called as the office was closing to check on him. That is when things started going downhill-as they always seem to do. It is always on a weekend or after hours when something changes. Chuck started throwing up his formula again and then threw up the Pedialyte®. Since we were concerned about dehydration, we decided to err on the side of caution and called the afterhours messaging service. When I spoke with the nurse she agreed that it did not sound like an emergency, but was concerned enough to advise us to take him to the emergency room where they could make sure he had enough fluids. I left my husband at home with Henry and at almost 11 pm went to the emergency room with Chuck, thinking he may need an IV for fluids. He slept on and off in his car seat as we waited for a doctor and had an x-ray of his abdomen to make sure there was no obstruction causing him to throw up.

The neonatologist and nurse were glad I had his discharge paperwork to easily see what his medical history was and both commented how amazing he looked for a 24 weeker. It took two tries but they were able to get an IV started to do some blood work, which showed he was slightly dehydrated but looked good otherwise. What the neonatologist was more concerned with was that his x-ray showed gas trapped in his intestines. With a normal healthy almost one year old, she said she would chalk it up to them being sick with a stomach bug and send them home to stay hydrated and wait for the gas to come out. However, given Chuck's intestinal history and her imaging limitations at that particular emergency room, she wanted to send him downtown to the children's hospital for further monitoring and tests to rule out a partial or complete bowel obstruction. That caught me off guard. I had thought that, worst case scenario, we would be in the ER for some IV fluids and be sent home a few hours later. Now all of a sudden I was calling my husband to let him know we were going downtown by ambulance, Chuck might possibly be very sick, and he was going to need to stay home from work with Henry.

Chuck slept on and off as I held him and we waited for the transfer paperwork. I asked the nurse which hospital we would be sent to and she told me that the emergency room was affiliated with a different hospital than the one the boys had been born. Not the one where all Chuck's surgeons and medical history was. She and I agreed that it made sense for him to be seen at his original hospital by his original surgeons since they knew him and his history. However, she believed that meant I would have to sign him out AMA, she would have to remove his IV, and I would have to drive him downtown and start the process all over in the emergency room of his original hospital. She hated to see him have to get another IV, as did I, but I felt strongly that it would make more sense in the long run for him to be seen by the doctors who knew him. Luckily the neonatologist came back a few minutes later to say that the first choice children's hospital was full and she could transfer us to Chuck's original hospital. We were all very glad that was the case.

Chuck and I went downtown by ambulance and arrived in the emergency room at 3 am. The neonatologist there agreed that Chuck could have a simple virus or he could have something much more serious and was glad we were there for monitoring. He ordered another x-ray to see if anything had changed with the gas in his intestine. They continued to give him fluids through the IV to keep him hydrated since they were not allowing him anything by mouth and he continued to sleep on and off. The ER was busy and it was 5 am by the time we finally settled into a small private ER room while the neonatologist consulted with Chuck's surgeon. I texted a few of Chuck's NICU nurses to let them know we were downstairs if any of them were working that day and could to come visit. They were sorry to hear Chuck was not feeling well, but they were glad we were in the best place for him. One let me know that in the ER, unlike the NICU, I could ask for the neonatologist or surgical attending if I had additional questions after we saw the fellow. That was good to know since I had not ever thought about who takes care of you in the ER. When the familiar face of Chuck's surgeon walked in at 6 am, I was so glad I gave him a hug. It was such a relief to feel like we were in the best place with people who knew Chuck and, regardless of what was wrong, he was going to be okay.

* * * * *

Hospitals and emergency rooms all have supplies for your baby that you might need while you are there. I ran out of diapers since I had only brought two in our diaper bag thinking we would be in the ER for a few hours. I was given diapers, wipes, and even borrowed a few toys while we were in the ER.

CHUCK'S SURGEON THOUGHT THAT IT WAS the right decision to come in for monitoring, but he was not overly nervous that there was an obstruction. He wanted us to stay a day or two to make sure the gas came out and Chuck was able to eat and drink normally. That sounded like a great plan to me given the alternative. Since the children's floor was equally busy, we waited in our ER room until noon before there was an empty room for us. I remembered from our time in the NICU that sugar water can be given on a pacifier before uncomfortable procedures and I asked for some. It helped to appease Chuck a bit since he was still on IV fluids but was not going to be given any formula for hours more, and it had been about 12 hours since he had kept anything down. The sugar water helped him feel as though he was eating something and made him happy. I was also able to leave him for a minute and run to the cafeteria to get a sandwich since I had not eaten since dinner the night before and it was by then early afternoon. I also had not slept at all the previous night because we were at the ER and in an ambulance or the night before that because Chuck was waking feeling crummy and I had spent the night on his floor to help him get back to sleep. It was difficult for me to hold his hand and help him sleep or play with him in any position but standing because of the height of the crib so I was getting pretty tired.

A little while after we were able to move to a room on the children's floor, Chuck's surgeon came to check on him again. I told him he had been very gassy, which I hoped was a sign that his body reacted to the bug by holding gas and making him feel yucky and was now getting a little better. He agreed and said we could try giving him some formula and if he kept it down he could possibly be discharged that evening and not be required to stay overnight. That was great news. Chuck did great keeping down a few ounces of formula, and a few hours later he was allowed to have some more. After that his surgeon felt confident it was just a stomach virus after all. We now knew that because of his intestinal history, Chuck may react differently than other kids to stomach viruses. My husband and Henry came and picked us up when Chuck was discharged late that evening, and we stopped at the ER on the way home for me to get my car. As soon as we got home we put both boys in bed and I immediately went to bed as well. The next day I was able to get in some naps when the boys napped to catch up on 48 hours of missed sleep. Chuck continued to slowly feel better and was completely back to normal within a few days.

* * * * *

We had a follow up visit with the Pedi Surg attending a week after our hospital stay and he agreed that unless there was an absolute emergency and time was of the essence, Chuck would ideally always be seen at his original hospital and by his original surgeons for anything remotely bowel related. That was good to know for the future. He also let us know that any bowel movement changes Chuck showed, either 1/3 less or 3x more, would be reasons to have him seen. We continued to chart Chuck's bowel movements with a check mark on a monthly calendar until he was 19 months old to make sure he was still within his norm.

* * * * *

Checking in with your original team of doctors and specialists, if possible, is always very helpful. There were different things to be aware of at different ages and I was always glad when we were seen by one of their original team.

* * * * *

It was helpful that friends and family members did not treat Chuck's visit back to the hospital as the end of the world. I was trying to stay calm and think positively, and it helped that no one around us freaked out.

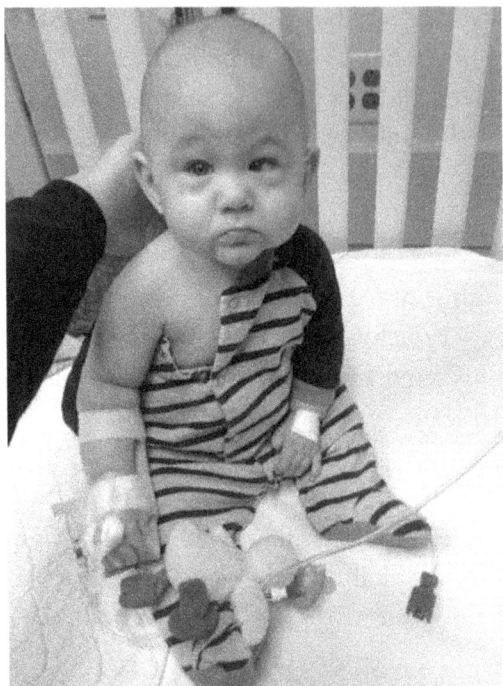

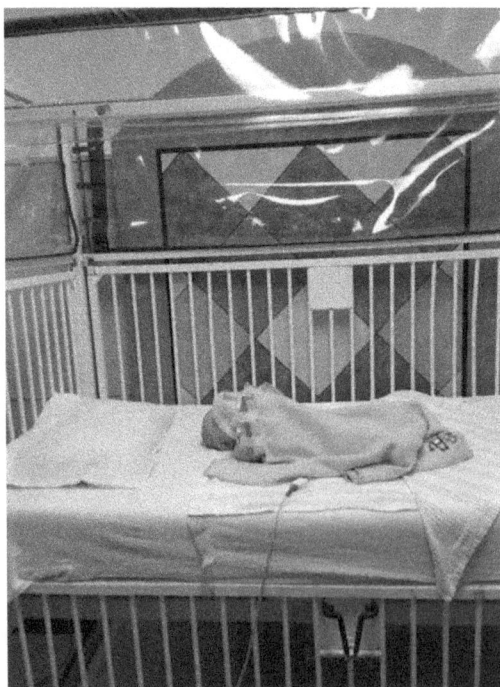

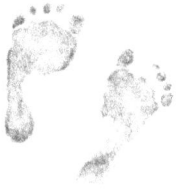

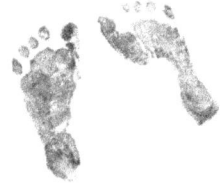

Helmets

ONE MORE THING WE ACCOMPLISHED AT Chuck's follow up appointment with his surgeon after his hospital visit was getting a second opinion concerning him needing a helmet. Since he had come home with the oxygen monitor, we were able to tell he sated best lying on his right side and we put him on that side to sleep. Unfortunately that, coupled with the length of time he had to stay on his back following his surgeries, led to him having a fairly noticeable asymmetrically flat head (plagiocephaly and brachycephaly). As much as the nurses tried to change his position while he was in the NICU, they could only do so much since he was not able to be on his stomach for months. As much as we did tummy time and repositioned him during naps, eventually letting him sleep on his tummy during naps, and repositioned him throughout the night, the shape of his head was not rounding out very much.

Although our pediatrician agreed it was noticeable and that a helmet was an option, he believed once Chuck had a normal amount of hair it would not be noticeable (although he may never want to shave his head completely). I was on the fence for two months following his discontinuation of the oxygen before we saw his surgeon for the follow up and asked his opinion. On one hand, I felt that anything purely aesthetic was not worth doing-the boys had been through enough and we did not need one more thing. But on the other hand, I did not want him to be a teenager and shave his head and be disappointed with the shape and that we could have given him a treatment to fix it that he would not remember but we had not. I asked his surgeon, whose opinion I trusted very much, what he would do if Chuck was his baby. He said he would think of a helmet like orthodontic braces; if there was a noninvasive treatment to fix something, why not fix it. If Chuck was his baby, he would not hesitate to get a helmet.

We had already had a consultation with the orthotics office, and Chuck's initial measurements put him in the moderate range for brachycephaly and the severe range for plagiosephaly. He was on the older side to start a helmet since our initial appointment was when he was 12 months old, but since he was still only 8 months adjusted there was still some time to correct the shape. Our insurance had denied covering the $2500 helmet, and I thought that meant the problem was not as severe as we thought. However, I later learned almost everyone I knew who had a child who had a helmet was initially denied by their insurance regardless of their child's measurements. After we got Chuck's surgeon's opinion, we decided we would pay out of pocket for the helmet. But by the time we actually picked it up, the orthotics and our pediatrician's offices had resubmitted enough supporting paperwork that the insurance company ended up approving the cost. Although it was a pain (more for us than him), it was made more difficult with his glasses, and it definitely garnered some stares in public (especially when we went out with the helmet, the glasses, AND the eye patch!), he only had to wear the helmet for 3 months and it made a huge difference. I am very glad we decided to do it, and I think he will be also when he is older.

* * * * *

Many preemies and micro preemies (in addition to some full term babies) have to wear helmets. Lots of tummy time from the very beginning can help to fix or avoid a helmet, but sometimes it cannot be avoided. Everyone I know who has a child who has had a helmet has said it is much harder on the parents than the child. Over the course of a few days the helmet wearing time increases until it is worn 23 hours a day. During the hour off (usually bath time) the helmet is washed with alcohol and dried. We used a hypoallergenic body wash during that time and an unscented cream for his head and were super lucky that his skin had zero problems. He had to wear it during the hot humid summer, and he runs hot to begin with, therefore, we did have to turn up the air conditioning in our house and dress him lighter than we normally would have to try to counteract the extra warmth the helmet gave him. His head would be smelly when we took the helmet off every day, and the helmet did acquire a smell all of its own (even with the alcohol bath every day), but he was still cute as a button and it was totally worth it. Of all the information about helmets I have seen, I have not read of a parent who got their child one and regretted the decision. If you are on the fence, I would get the opinion of a medical professional you trust and not fear the helmet.

* * * * *

All babies are cute and get stared at when you leave the house so do not give it a second thought if your baby has extra "stuff" and gets stared at in public! We did not go anywhere except the doctor's while Chuck was on oxygen because it was too cumbersome, but later on he sported glasses, an eye patch, and a helmet so we definitely got some looks. A few times I heard a mother telling her child the baby had "hurt his eye" or "hurt his head" when the child had asked what was wrong with Chuck. Chuck, however, was completely oblivious and loved going out. We simply put blinders on unless someone asked us a question directly and went about our business. There is always a child with a more severe challenge than yours; therefore, it is important not to hide because your child needs extra "stuff".

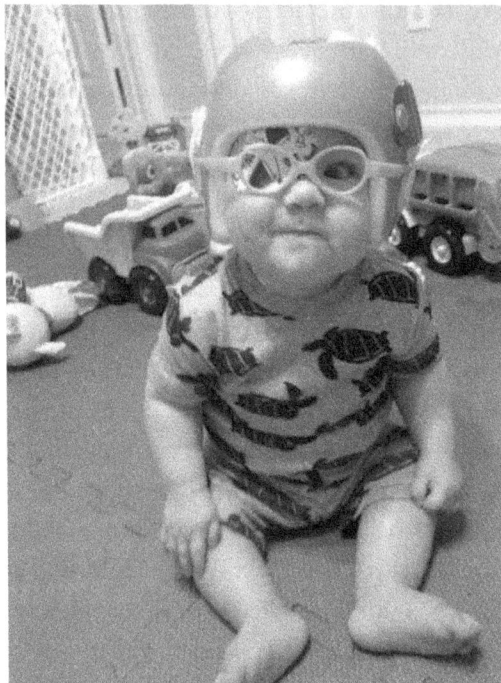

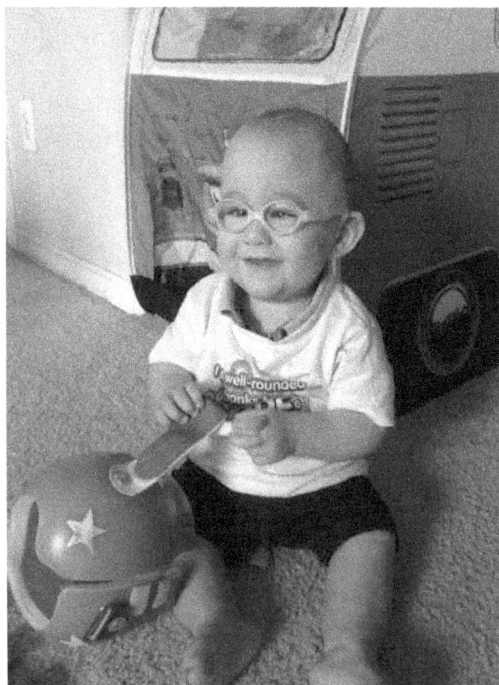

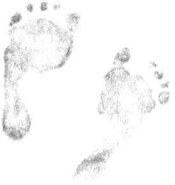

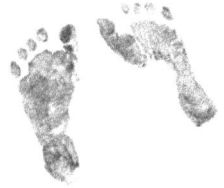

We Made it Through the First Year!

BY THE TIME THEY WERE 12 MONTHS OLD, the boys were starting to really enjoy going out into the world, becoming more mobile on their own, crawling and pulling up to walk along the couch, eating three meals a day with two snacks of a milk smoothie, and were done with bottles. We had introduced straw cups a few times a week starting at about 9 months old just for fun, and by the time the boys were 12 months they had no problem drinking out of them and did not miss their bottles when we took them away on their first birthday. They were starting to interact with each other, mostly in the form of random tackles that sort of looked like hugs. We were still working on sorting blocks, stacking rings, putting toys into other toys and containers, and basically playing appropriately with toys to strengthen and continue to improve their fine and gross motor skills.

* * * * *

At the boys' 12 month well baby checkup the pediatrician told us their calories should now come mainly from food with milk at meals. We decided on goat milk since I was able to find it with more calories and fat per serving than cow's milk. It made me nervous that for the first time we would be giving them food and then milk rather than milk and then food, since milk is much more calorie dense. I was worried about them being able to continue gaining weight well. To that end, we divided the ounces of milk recommended between their three meals and then used the rest as "snacks" in a smoothie with peanut butter, a banana per child, and coconut oil. We did this twice a day when they woke from naps, so that they had a calorically dense snack. They loved cheerios and goldfish, but those do not have very many calories and anything else was too messy to eat in the play room. We also incorporated a lot of avocado, cheese, and good oils into their meals (along with a ton of veggies and fruits). Luckily they were great eaters for the most part and continued to gain weight appropriately.

WE THREW THE BOYS A "ONE FISH, TWO FISH" themed first birthday party at our house and invited a few local family members, friends, and their NICU nurses. They each got to smash a cake, try ice cream, and play with new toys. It was fun for us to show their nurses how far they had come in a year. Other than my husband and me, these women had literally spent the most time with the boys, more than anyone else, and we loved that they could be a part of their first birthday because we would not have made it to that day without them. It was a day filled with emotions almost opposite of those the year before. When the boys were born we were scared, terrified really, and concerned about their survival and ability to lead a normal life. To see them at their first birthday happy, healthy, and almost caught up to their full term peers was truly a joyful day and we could not have asked for more.

* * * * *

We still, even with the boys being almost 2 years old, get a lot of questions because we have twins, because most people are not used to seeing a child so young wearing glasses, and because they are not the same size as their peers. The comments and questions we get run the gamut and can be rude, offensive, and completely inappropriate. Because I have twins I have people ask if they are identical, why one has glasses and the other does not, and how they were conceived. Because we have two boys, we are often told we should have another baby to ensure we have a girl. When someone asks their age, I get told a lot how small they are and sometimes asked their weight and height. It is not the best feeling to have someone guess they are months and months younger than they really are or exclaim again and again how small they are or how their child at so much younger weighed more or was taller. I answer questions honestly, for the most part. Yes, he wears glasses. No, they are not "play" (who does that to a baby or a toddler?) glasses, but he really does need them to see. Yes, I am aware his eyes look crossed, he does in fact have a lazy eye he needs surgically corrected. Yes, I realize they are small; they were born early and they are still catching up. Yes, they are twins. No, really, they are. Not all twins are identical. No, I do not have a favorite. Yes, I am very busy. No, we do not need to have more kids. No, we do not feel like we need to have another baby to have a girl. Yes, they are adorable.

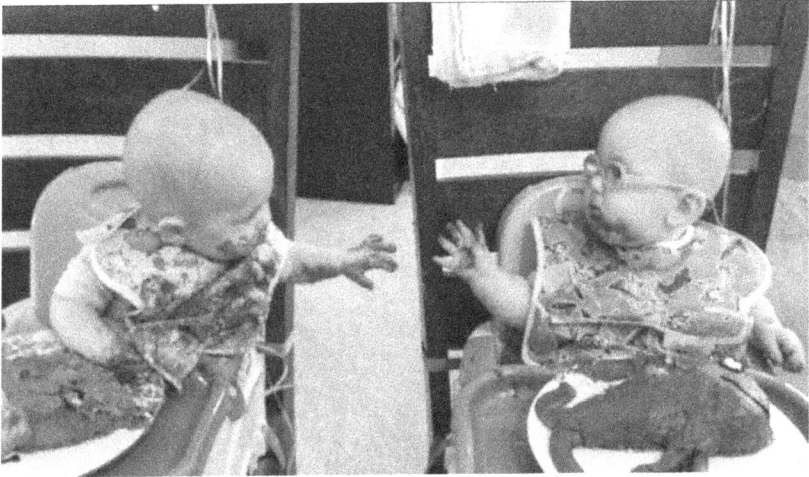

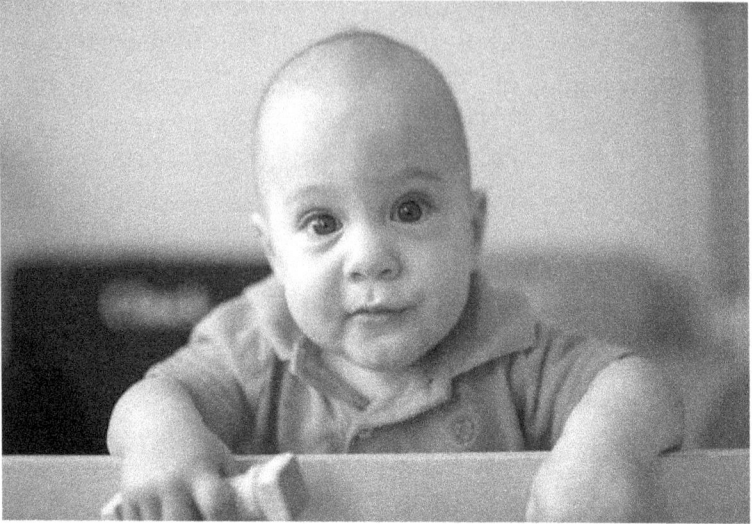

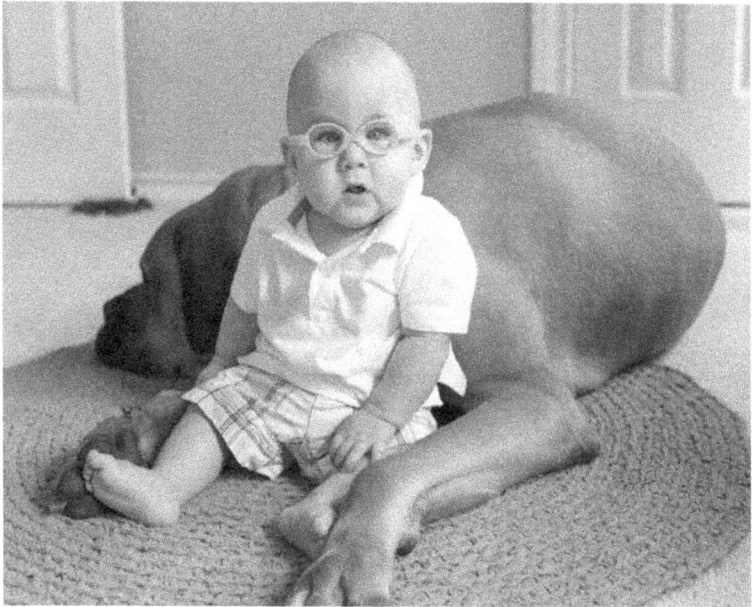

<u>Afterward</u>

EVEN NOW, AS THE BOYS ARE COUNTING DOWN the months until they turn 2 years old, we still get questions about how old they are and get some surprised looks since they are still small for their age and catching up in height and weight. Both boys were walking well by the time they were 16 months old and climbing, clapping, running and saying more words all the time when they were 19 months old. We cannot ask for more in terms of progress. We only see the pediatrician now for standard appointments. Chuck will have surgery in the spring to correct his lazy eyes, and he will continue to wear glasses and patches every day for the foreseeable future, but his ophthalmologist predicts a very positive outcome and a normal life regardless of the amount of depth perception he is able to achieve. None of our specialists are concerned with Chuck being at risk for Cerebral Palsy anymore, and although both boys are at higher risk for difficulties in school and ADHD, we are hopeful that their progress so far indicates that they will skirt by those problems as they have all the other things they were at a much higher risk for and have as of yet avoided. We are still very conscious of germs since the boys are more susceptible to more serious lung problems over the flu season and we have fewer playdates and activities with large groups during flu season even now. We continue to be very aware of issues that could involve Chuck's intestines. We continue to work on milestones and improving the boys' development just like other kids.

Our doctors tell us it is reasonable that the boys could catch up to their peers around their second birthday. Walking at 15 months, sleeping in toddler beds at 16 months old and saying close to 20 words at 21 months old all speak to the very real possibility the boys will look just like every other toddler soon. I have made a first year photo book for both boys so that someday, when they are old enough, they can understand how they came into the world. They will be able to see their hospital pod, their nurses, and everything it took to get them home. Statistically, coming out the other side of this journey with two healthy and happy boys puts us in the lucky 20% of 24 weekers. We are enjoying every day with our boys and look forward to their bright futures.

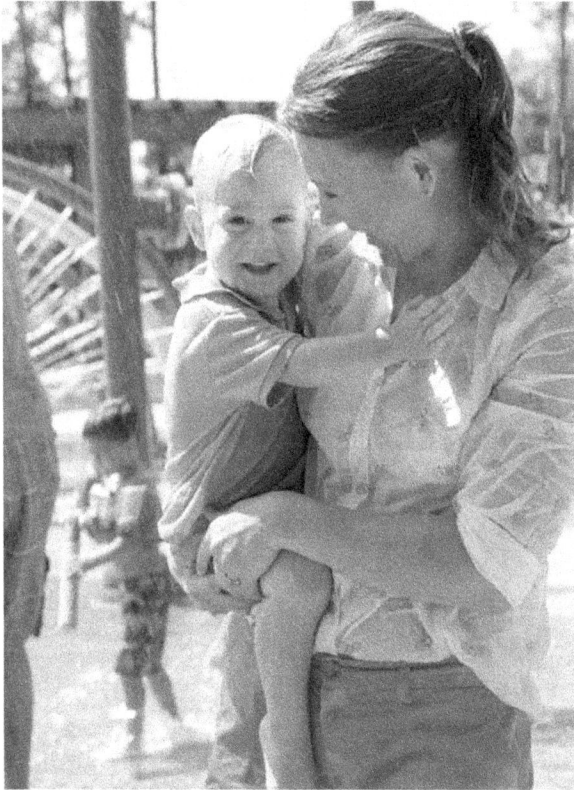

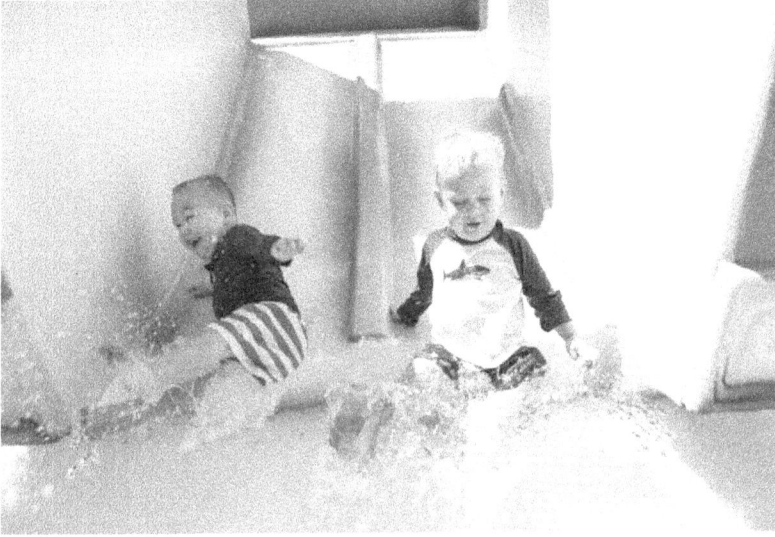

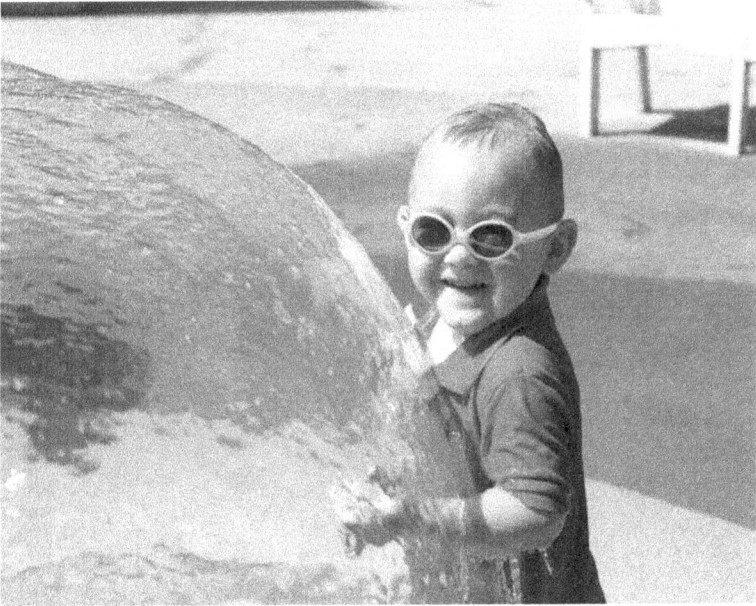

Tiny

<u>Sources</u>

Luke, Barbara, and Eberlein, Tamara. *When You're Expecting Twins, Triplets or Quads.* HarperCollins, 2011.

March of Dimes, March of Dimes Foundation. Web, 2015.

Facts & Figures. Preemie Help: Everything Preterm Birth. Web, 2009-2013.

Hope and Healing. CaringBridge. Web, 1997-2015.

Gephart, Sheila M, RN, BSN; McGrath, Jacqueline, PhD, RN; Effkin, Judith, PhD, RN; Halpern, Melissa D, PhD. *Necrotizing Entercolitis Risk.* Adv Neonatal Care. 2012 April; 12(2) 77-89.

Kim, Jae H, MD, PhD, FRCPC, FAAP. *An Exclusive Human Milk Diet Can Reduce Necrotizing Entercolitis.* Babies with NEC, Web. June 4th, 2010.

Manzoni P, et all. *Human milk feeding prevents retinopathy of prematurity (ROP) in preterm VLBW neonates.* Early Human Dev. Web. 2013 Jun; 89suppl 1:S64-8.

Griggs, Paul B, MD. *Retinopathy of Prematurity.* MedLine Plus. U.S. National Library of Medicine, National Institues of Health. Web. 26 April 2013.

Larimer, Krisanne. *Kangaroo Care Benefits.* Prematurity. Web. 1999.

Culver, Ashley. *Vanderbilt study shows mother's voice improves hospitalization and feeding in preemies.* Vanderbuilt University. Web. 17 Feb 2014.

Infant-Food and Feeding. American Association of Pediatrics. Web. 2014.

Clayton, Heather, PhD, MPH; Li, Ruowei, MD, PhD; Scanlon, Kelley, PhD, RD. *Prevalence and Reasons for Introducing Infants Early to Solid Foods: Variations by Milk Feeding Type.* Pediatrics, 25 Mar 2013. Web.

Thank You

Thank you so much to my partner in this journey, my husband, Pete. We make the best team and I love you.

Thank you Jonathon Wolfer for your expertise, time and talent.

Thank you to Tiny Diver for taking on my project.

Thank you Jordyn Hagar, Kim Hegar and Amanda Tobey for your editing and feedback. Your time and encouragement meant so much.

Thank you to everyone that, over the last year and a half, ever said, "You should write a book!"

Most importantly, thank you to the two boys who made me a mom. I love you more than you will ever know.

"You're braver than you believe, and stronger than you seem, and smarter than you think"

A.A. Milne

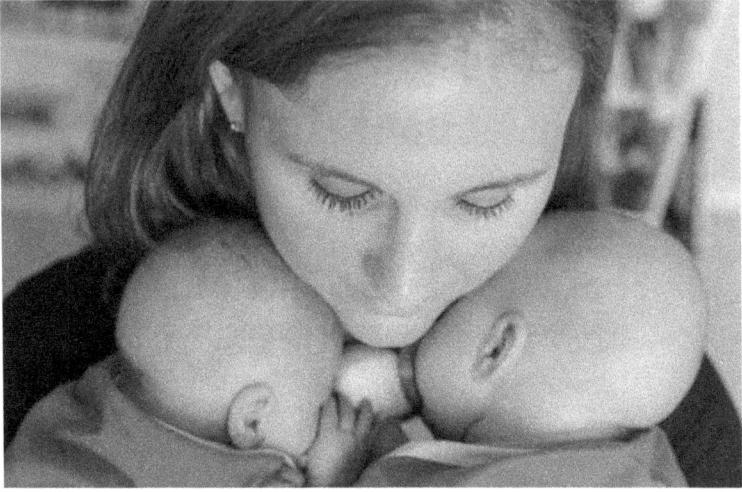

Originally from the East coast, Joanna graduated cum laude from Saint Anselm College with a degree in Biochemistry. She currently lives in Spring, Texas, with her husband and twin boys. She loves her exhausting job as a full time mom.

But Mighty

Tiny

Tiny

www.ingramcontent.com/pod-product-compliance
Lightning Source LLC
LaVergne TN
LVHW011154080426
835508LV00007B/401